ANTI-ANGIOGENESIS STRATEGIES IN CANCER THERAPIES

ANTI-ANGIOGENESIS STRATEGIES IN CANCER THERAPIES

Edited by

SHAKER A. MOUSA
The Pharmaceutical Research Institute
Albany College of Pharmacy and Health Sciences
Rensselaer, New York, United States

PAUL J. DAVIS
Department of Medicine, Albany Medical College
Albany, New York, United States
The Pharmaceutical Research Institute
Albany College of Pharmacy and Health Sciences
Rensselaer, New York, United States

ELSEVIER

Amsterdam • Boston • Heidelberg • London
New York • Oxford • Paris • San Diego
San Francisco • Singapore • Sydney • Tokyo

Academic Press is an imprint of Elsevier

Academic Press is an imprint of Elsevier
125 London Wall, London EC2Y 5AS, United Kingdom
525 B Street, Suite 1800, San Diego, CA 92101-4495, United States
50 Hampshire Street, 5th Floor, Cambridge, MA 02139, United States
The Boulevard, Langford Lane, Kidlington, Oxford OX5 1GB, United Kingdom

Notices

Knowledge and best practice in this field are constantly changing. As new research and experience
broaden our understanding, changes in research methods, professional practices, or medical treatment
may become necessary.

Practitioners and researchers must always rely on their own experience and knowledge in evaluating and
using any information, methods, compounds, or experiments described herein. In using such information or methods they should be mindful of their own safety and the safety of others, including parties
for whom they have a professional responsibility.

To the fullest extent of the law, neither the Publisher nor the authors, contributors, or editors, assume
any liability for any injury and/or damage to persons or property as a matter of products liability,
negligence or otherwise, or from any use or operation of any methods, products, instructions, or ideas
contained in the material herein.

Library of Congress Cataloging-in-Publication Data
A catalog record for this book is available from the Library of Congress

British Library Cataloguing-in-Publication Data
A catalogue record for this book is available from the British Library

ISBN: 978-0-12-802576-5

For information on all Academic Press publications
visit our website at https://www.elsevier.com/

  Working together
to grow libraries in
developing countries

www.elsevier.com • www.bookaid.org

Publisher: Mica Haley
Acquisition Editor: Kristine Jones
Editorial Project Manager: Molly McLaughlin
Production Project Manager: Julia Haynes
Designer: Mark Rogers

Typeset by Thomson Digital

CONTENTS

LIST OF CONTRIBUTORS

Maii Abu Taleb
The Pharmaceutical Research Institute, Albany College of Pharmacy and Health Sciences, Rensselaer, NY, United States

Dhruba J. Bharali
The Pharmaceutical Research Institute, Albany College of Pharmacy and Health Sciences, Rensselaer, NY, United States

Noureldien H.E. Darwish
The Pharmaceutical Research Institute, Albany College of Pharmacy and Health Sciences, Rensselaer, NY, United States; Faculty of Medicine, Mansoura University, Mansoura, Egypt

Paul J. Davis
Department of Medicine, Albany Medical College, Albany, NY, United States; The Pharmaceutical Research Institute, Albany College of Pharmacy and Health Sciences, Rensselaer, NY, United States

Matthew Leinung
Department of Medicine, Albany Medical College, Albany, NY, United States

Shaker A. Mousa
The Pharmaceutical Research Institute, Albany College of Pharmacy and Health Sciences, Rensselaer, NY, United States

Vandhana Muralidharan-Chari
The Pharmaceutical Research Institute, Albany College of Pharmacy and Health Sciences, Rensselaer, NY, United States

Mehdi Rajabi
The Pharmaceutical Research Institute, Albany College of Pharmacy and Health Sciences, Rensselaer, NY, United States

Domenico Ribatti
Department of Basic Medical Sciences, Neurosciences and Sensory Organs, University of Bari Medical School; National Cancer Institute "Giovanni Paolo II", Bari, Italy

Thangirala Sudha
The Pharmaceutical Research Institute, Albany College of Pharmacy and Health Sciences, Rensselaer, NY, United States

Angelo Vacca
Department of Biomedical Sciences, and Human Oncology, Section of Internal Medicine and Clinical Oncology, University of Bari Medical School, Bari, Italy

Murat Yalcin
The Pharmaceutical Research Institute, Albany College of Pharmacy and Health Sciences, Rensselaer, NY, United States; Department of Physiology, Veterinary Medicine Faculty, Uludag University, Bursa, Turkey

Introduction

The requirement of aggressive cancers for rapidly growing blood vessels with unique structures [1,2] has rendered anti-angiogenesis [3] a highly attractive adjunct to standard chemotherapy or has led to its consideration as single-agent treatment. Anti-angiogenesis has been tested against a spectrum of solid tumors, including breast [4], ovary [5], prostate [6], hepatocellular carcinoma [7], lung cancers [8], and colon [9], among others.

However, reviews of anti-angiogenic therapy in cancer conclude that this approach to-date has been disappointing [10–14]. Redundancy and upregulation of compensatory pro-angiogenesis pathways are a hallmark of tumor cell defenses in general and, not unexpectedly, our appreciation of the scope of mechanisms of tumor refractoriness to anti-angiogenesis continues to increase [15–18]. This has led to consideration of new directions in interventions in cancer-related blood vessel formation. Such new directions include combinations of anti-angiogenic agents [12], DNA-based immunotherapy directed at vasculature [19,20], anti-inflammation [21], anti-platelet therapy [22], and novel small molecules that serve to regulate the functions of multiple angiogenic factors [23,24]. Additionally, certain angiogenesis pathways, such as the integrin $\alpha v\beta 3$ receptor complex might serve as a novel targeting strategy for imaging and targeted delivery for a nanoencapsulated payload of various chemotherapies (Chapter 11).

In this book, we summarize a number of mechanisms for limitations of anti-angiogenic interventions in cancer and have assembled reviews of a panel of strategies that may serve to improve effectiveness of anti-angiogenic interventions, alone, in cancer or in combination with chemotherapy.

REFERENCES

[1] Dvorak HF, Weaver VM, Tlsty TD, Bergers G. Tumor microenvironment and progression. J Surg Oncol 2011;103(6):468–74.

[2] Nagy JA, Chang SH, Shih SC, Dvorak AM, Dvorak HF. Heterogeneity of the tumor vasculature. Semin Thromb Hemost 2010;36(3):321–31.

[3] Abdollahi A, Folkman J. Evading tumor evasion: current concepts and perspectives of anti-angiogenic cancer therapy. Drug Resist Updat 2010;13(1–2):16–28.

[4] Lohmann AE, Chia S. Patients with metastatic breast cancer using bevacizumab as a treatment: is there still a role for it? Curr Treat Options Oncol 2012;13(2):249–62.

[5] Eskander RN, Tewari KS. Incorporation of anti-angiogenesis therapy in the management of advanced ovarian carcinoma--mechanistics, review of phase III randomized clinical trials, and regulatory implications. Gynecol Oncol 2014;132(2):496–505.

[6] Bilusic M, Wong YN. Anti-angiogenesis in prostate cancer: knocked down but not out. Asian J Androl 2014;16(3):372–7.

[7] Sun H, Zhu MS, Wu WR, Shi XD, Xu LB. Role of anti-angiogenesis therapy in the management of hepatocellular carcinoma: the jury is still out. World J Hepatol 2014;6(12):830–5.

[8] Ellis PM. Anti-angiogenesis in personalized therapy of lung cancer. Adv Exp Med Biol 2016;893:91–126.

[9] Marien KM, Croons V, Martinet W, De Loof H, Ung C, Waelput W, Scherer SJ, Kockx MM, De Meyer GR. Predictive tissue biomarkers for bevacizumab-containing therapy in metastatic colorectal cancer: an update. Expert Rev Mol Diagn 2015;15(3):399–414.

[10] Shojaei F. Anti-angiogenesis therapy in cancer: current challenges and future perspectives. Cancer Lett 2012;320(2):130–7.

[11] Bellou S, Pentheroudakis G, Murphy C, Fotsis T. Anti-angiogenesis in cancer therapy: Hercules and hydra. Cancer Lett 2013;338(2):219–28.

[12] Wang Z, Dabrosin C, Yin X, Fuster MM, Arreola A, Rathmell WK, Generali D, Nagaraju GP, El-Rayes B, Ribatti D, Chen YC, Honoki K, Fujii H, Georgakilas AG, Nowsheen S, Amedei A, Niccolai E, Amin A, Ashraf SS, Helferich B, Yang X, Guha G, Bhakta D, Ciriolo MR, Aquilano K, Chen S, Halicka D, Mohammed SI, Azmi AS, Bilsland A, Keith WN, Jensen LD. Broad targeting of angiogenesis for cancer prevention and therapy. Semin Cancer Biol 2015;35:S224–43.

[13] Mitamura T, Gourley C, Sood AK. Prediction of anti-angiogenesis escape. Gynecol Oncol 2016;141(1):80–5.

[14] Ye W. The complexity of translating anti-angiogenesis therapy from basic science to the clinic. Dev Cell 2016;37(2):114–25.

[15] Giuliano S, Pages G. Mechanisms of resistance to anti-angiogenesis therapies. Biochimie 2013;95(6):1110–9.

[16] Ribatti D. Tumor refractoriness to anti-VEGF therapy. Oncotarget 2016.

[17] Huijbers EJ, van Beijnum JR, Thijssen VL, Sabrkhany S, Nowak-Sliwinska P, Griffioen AW. Role of the tumor stroma in resistance to anti-angiogenic therapy. Drug Resist Updat 2016;25:26–37.

[18] Pinto MC, Sotomayor P, Carrasco-Avino G, Corvalan AH, Owen GI. Escaping antiangiogenic therapy: strategies employed by cancer cells. Int J Mol Sci 2016;17(9.).

[19] Ugel S, Facciponte JG, De Sanctis F, Facciabene A. Targeting tumor vasculature: expanding the potential of DNA cancer vaccines. Cancer Immunol Immunother 2015;64(10):1339–48.

[20] Wagner SC, Ichim TE, Ma H, Szymanski J, Perez JA, Lopez J, Bogin V, Patel AN, Marincola FM, Kesari S. Cancer anti-angiogenesis vaccines: is the tumor vasculature antigenically unique? J Transl Med 2015;13:340.

[21] Ribatti D, Crivellato E, Vacca A. Inflammation and antiangiogenesis in cancer. Curr Med Chem 2012;19(7):955–60.

[22] Yan M, Lesyk G, Radziwon-Balicka A, Jurasz P. Pharmacological regulation of platelet factors that influence tumor angiogenesis. Semin Oncol 2014;41(3):370–7.

[23] Mousa SA, Lin HY, Tang HY, Hercbergs A, Luidens MK, Davis PJ. Modulation of angiogenesis by thyroid hormone and hormone analogues: implications for cancer management. Angiogenesis 2014;17(3):463–9.

[24] Davis PJ, Sudha T, Lin HY, Mousa SA. Thyroid hormone, hormone analogs, and angiogenesis. Compr Physiol 2015;6(1):353–62.

CHAPTER 1

Angiogenesis and Anti-Angiogenesis Strategies in Cancer

Shaker A. Mousa and Paul J. Davis

Contents

Anti-Angiogenesis Strategies in Cancer Therapies
http://dx.doi.org/10.1016/B978-0-12-802576-5.00001-2

PROCESS OF ANGIOGENESIS

Angiogenesis is a complex process in which endogenous local or systemic chemical signals coordinate functions of endothelial cells and smooth muscle cells. Both repair of damaged blood vessels and the formation of new blood vessels can be achieved with these signals. Another set of chemical signals, angiogenesis inhibitors (Table 1.1), may systematically disrupt blood vessel formation or support removal of existing vessels, for example, at the conclusion of an inflammatory response. In the setting of homeostasis, the stimulating and inhibiting chemical signals are balanced and blood vessels form only as they are needed.

Angiogenic support is critical to growth and spread of cancer. Growth of localized tumors beyond a few millimeters in size

Table 1.1 Selected list of endogenous angiogenesis inhibitors and mechanisms of action

Endogenous angiogenesis inhibitors	Mechanisms
Soluble VEGF-1	Decoy receptors for VEGF-B
Angiostatin	Suppress EC adhesion, migration, proliferation
Thrombospondin-1 and -2	Suppress EC adhesion, migration, proliferation
Angiopoietin-2	Oppose angiopoietin-1
Platelet factor-4	Inhibit bFGF (FGF2) and VEGF binding
Endostatin	Suppress EC adhesion, migration, proliferation
Anti-thrombin III fragment	Suppress EC adhesion, migration, proliferation
Osteopontin	Serve as ligand for integrin binding
Collagen	Substrate for MMPs
Kininogen domains	Suppress EC adhesion, migration, proliferation
Tissue factor pathways inhibitor	Antagonist for tissue factor

Abbreviations: bFGF, basic fibroblast growth factor; EC, endothelial cell; MMP, matrix metalloproteinase; VEGF, vascular endothelial growth factor.

requires local angiogenesis. Tumor cells generate new blood vessel formation by releasing proangiogenic chemical signals. Normal cells proximal to cancer cells may also support a proangiogenic response via signaling molecules. Local neovascularization supplies growing tumors with oxygen and essential nutrients, supports tumor extension and invasion into nearby normal tissue, and is essential to distant metastasis [1,2].

ANGIOGENESIS IN CANCER

As in normal tissues, tumor tissue is unable to grow or metastasize locally or systemically without angiogenic support. The vessels supply oxygen and nutrients required for growth [2]. The hypoxic tumor cell, for example, at the center of a typically spheroid cancer in situ, will not divide. This state may serve as a survival mechanism when such cells are exposed to therapeutic measures—radiation or certain chemotherapeutic agents—that disrupt DNA only when it is undergoing division.

The walls of blood vessels are endothelial cells that divide and migrate in response to local signals. The sequential steps of new blood vessel creation include activation of the endothelial cell wall of an existing small blood vessel (capillary), secretion of metalloproteinase enzymes that degrade the proteinaceous extracellular matrix (surrounding tissue), invasion of the matrix, and then cell division. String-like lattices of new endothelial cells organize into hollow tubes, resulting in new blood vessel networks that enable surrounding (cancer) tissue growth [2–4].

In nonmalignant tissues, endothelial cells are largely dormant. In growing cancers, endothelial cells are vigorously active. When needed in normal tissues or organs, new capillary growth is closely regulated by release of factors that activate endothelial cells and factors (Table 1.1) that are inhibitory [2,3]. Such a balance is less apparent in cancers, where anti-angiogenic factor production is of course reduced.

Among many proteins, known to activate endothelial cell growth and motility, are angiogenin, epidermal growth factor (EGF), estrogen, fibroblast growth factors (acidic and basic), interleukin 8, prostaglandin E1 and E2, tumor necrosis factor-α, vascular endothelial growth factor (VEGF), and granulocyte colony-stimulating factor [5]. VEGF and basic fibroblast growth factor (bFGF; FGF2) are particularly important to tumor angiogenesis [2,3], but the redundancy of (other) proangiogenic factors helps explain the suboptimal effectiveness to-date in oncology of pharmacological inhibitors of single endogenous angiogenic agents. We have pointed out that physiological concentrations of thyroid hormone are proangiogenic by multiple mechanisms [6] and have raised the possibility that this hormone is a model of nonprotein stimulators of angiogenesis that may contribute to clinical resistance to anti-angiogenesis drugs.

Naturally occurring angiogenesis inhibitors are angiostatin, endostatin, interferons, interleukins 1 and 12, tissue inhibitor of metalloproteinases, and retinoic acid [2,3,7,8]. Additional factors are included in Table 1.1. Pharmaceutical models of angiogenesis inhibitors are antibodies to VEGF and the anti-cancer tyrosine kinase inhibitors (TKIs) that block activities/functions of growth factor receptors relevant to angiogenesis.

Tumor-related angiogenesis is an important factor in metastasis. Highly vascular tumors have higher likelihoods of metastasis and poorer prognoses. A full blood vessel network appears to be associated with tumor cell shedding. Matrix metalloproteinase (MMP) enzymes support both angiogenesis and metastasis in that they break down the microenvironment of tumors (extracellular matrix), permitting tumor growth, expansion of tumor circulation, and space for shed cells [2,4].

In the absence of vascular growth factors, endothelial cells in major blood vessels unrelated to cancer divide at 1000-day intervals [9], a rate that does not support cancer growth. The phase of rapid growth in cancers and metastasis requires profound angiogenesis and lymphangiogenesis [10], and each stimulatory component of angiogenesis that supports tumor growth is a potential target for new cancer therapies. Understandably, anti-angiogenic pharmaceutical development has become an essential component of the anti-cancer drug industry. However, improved pharmaceutical strategies are required if targeting of tumor blood supplies is to achieve the clinical effectiveness that our improved understanding of mechanisms of angiogenesis has predicted.

STRATEGIES

In general, four strategies are used by investigators to design anti-angiogenesis agents:

1. inhibition of actions of endogenous factors that stimulate the formation of blood vessels;
2. identification and exploitation of natural inhibitors of angiogenesis;
3. inhibition of molecules that facilitate invasion of surrounding tissue by tumor-related blood vessels; and
4. incapacitation of actively dividing endothelial cells.

The best understood components of angiogenesis may not be optimal single pharmacologic targets because of the redundancy in cancer-related angiogenesis of vascular growth factors and the heterogeneity of structure of tumor blood supply. For example, VEGF-dependent and -independent vessels may coexist within a given tumor [11,12]. Such observations encourage multifactor treatment regimens that require several types of anti-angiogenic therapy or a combination of anti-angiogenic drug therapy with cytotoxic anti-tumor therapy. An interesting model in this regard has been the integrin inhibitor, cilengitide. Cilengitide targets both tumor cells and activated, tumor-related vasculature [13] because both express cell surface integrins bearing the cilengitide target, an Arg-Gly-Asp (RGD) recognition site. Results of clinical trials of cilengitide against glioblastoma [14] have been disappointing [15,16], despite the agent's targeting of both tumor and endothelial cells. The agent has also been tested against other tumors [17]. The RGD recognition site is of importance to the interaction of the plasma membrane integrin with extracellular matrix (ECM) proteins, but this site may not be essential to tumor biology. On the other hand, we now know that there are small molecule receptors on a particular integrin ($\alpha v\beta 3$) that in a highly complex manner regulate transcription of vascular growth factor genes and of certain cancer cell survival genes. Thyroid hormone is one such small molecule that acts on a specific integrin in a manner far more complex than the activity of cilengitide on multiple integrins [18,19]. Other small molecules with receptors on integrin $\alpha v\beta 3$ include androgen [20] and a stilbene, resveratrol [21]. Thus, specific integrins and very specific domains on specific integrins may be candidate anti-cancer drug targets that affect multiple functions of endothelial cells and of cancer cells.

CURRENT EXAMPLES OF CANCER TREATMENT AGENTS THAT BLOCK ANGIOGENESIS

Angiogenesis inhibitors are designed to prevent the formation of new blood vessels. Such action may stop or slow the growth and spread of tumors. This may not eradicate tumors unless the therapeutic anti-angiogenic agent also induces dissolution of extant blood vessels serving the cancer. For optimal efficacy, a combination of prospective anti-angiogenesis and tumor cell chemotherapy may be required. The US Food and Drug Administration (FDA) has approved a number of angiogenesis inhibitors for the treatment of cancers, as listed here and in Table 1.2:

1. thalidomide for the treatment for multiple myeloma (MM) and other types of cancer;
2. lenalidomide for the treatment of MM and a specific type of myelodysplastic syndrome (MDS);

Table 1.2 FDA-approved vascular growth factor inhibitors

Generic name	Trade name	FDA-approved indication
Bevacizumab	Avastin	Colorectal, non-small cell lung, and glioblastoma multiforme
Sorafenib	Nexavar	Renal cell and hepatocellular carcinoma
Sunitinib	Sutent	Renal cell and gastrointestinal carcinoma
Pazopanib	Votrient	Renal cell carcinoma

3. bevacizumab, a monoclonal antibody to VEGF, for colorectal cancer, kidney cancer, breast cancer, lung cancer, and other types of cancer;
4. sunitinib, a TKI, for kidney cancer, gastrointestinal stromal tumor; and
5. sorafenib, a TKI, for kidney and liver cancer.

SIDE EFFECTS OF ANGIOGENESIS INHIBITORS

Angiogenesis inhibitors can interfere with wound healing [22,23]. These agents may cause hypertension [22].

Inherent and acquired resistance to angiogenesis inhibitors has been described [12,24,25], as have induction of tumor invasiveness and prothrombotic adverse events [22]. Possible mechanisms of resistance include selection of clonal tumor cell populations with capacities to upregulate alternative proangiogenic pathways, selection of cells with increased invasiveness, and cells that are hypoxia-insensitive. In addition, lack of thoroughly validated predictive biomarkers has limited the capacity to stratify cancer patients and to monitor tumor progression and response to the therapy.

ANGIOGENESIS AND ANGIOGENESIS INHIBITORS: POTENTIAL ANTI-CANCER THERAPEUTIC EFFICACY

Targeting of VEGF

Unless tumors induce sufficient vascularization, they are unable to grow to a mass greater than 2–3 mm^3; this limitation reflects insufficiency of diffusion to meet oxygen and glucose requirements of tumor cells. Thus, successful anti-angiogenesis at a tumor site has the capacity to arrest tumor growth without necessarily interfering with cell viability. An agent that is able to promote devascularization of a tumor, that is, remove existing blood vessels, will cause tumor cell necrosis. VEGF is the most extensively studied endogenous proangiogenic factor and, as a result, much research attention

Table 1.3 VEGF signaling inhibitors

Antibodies (anti-VEGFR-2) VEGF trap RTKs with anti-VEGF properties	Ramucirumab Aflibercept Axitinib Cediranib Regorafenib Semaxanib Torceranib Vandetanib Brivanib

Abbreviations: RTKs, Receptor tyrosine kinases; VEGF, vascular endothelial growth factor; VEGFR, VEGF receptor.

has been devoted pharmacologically to inhibition of VEGF action, for example, interference with VEGF signaling (Table 1.3). VEGF is an endothelial cell-specific mitogen and an angiogenic inducer. It is essential for developmental angiogenesis, for bone formation, and for female reproductive functions. Humanized VEGF monoclonal antibody (rhuMab VEGF) is in clinical trials as a treatment for various solid tumors. In Phase II clinical studies of patients with colorectal and lung cancer, anti-VEGF in conjunction with standard chemotherapy has shown efficacy [26,27]. Additionally, anti-VEGF strategies have been shown to be effective in various ocular neovascularization disorders [28,29]. Small molecule inhibitors of receptor tyrosine kinases (RTKs) (Table 1.3) may also interfere with VEGF action at its receptor (VEGFR).

ADDITIONAL ANTI-ANGIOGENESIS STRATEGIES IN CANCERS

Kininostatin

Studied in the chick chorioallantoic membrane (CAM) model, domain 5 (D5) of high molecular weight kininogen has been shown to inhibit endothelial cell migration toward a vitronectin cue and to decrease endothelial cell proliferation and angiogenesis. D5 contains a peptide sequence that is migration-specific and another sequence that inhibits only proliferation. The contributions of kininogen to angiogenesis have also been confirmed with an inhibitory monoclonal antibody [30].

Alpha 3 Chain of Type IV Collagen

Collagen is an essential component of the scaffolding of basement membranes and the noncollagenous domains of collagen have been found to have potent anti-angiogenic activity. We have shown that a specific peptide comprising residues 185–203 of the noncollagenous domain (NC1) of the alpha 3 (Type IV) collagen chain has a variety of biological activities, including inhibition of neutrophil activation, support of tumor cell adhesion and chemotaxis, and inhibition of tumor cell proliferation [31]. Peptides from the NC1 domain have shown important anti-angiogenic activity [32].

Matrix Metalloproteinases

Matrix metalloproteinases (MMPs) are zinc-dependent endopeptidases that degrade ECM proteins—collagen, laminin, and fibronectin—during the process of cancer invasion and metastasis. MMPs are produced primarily by reactive stromal and inflammatory cells surrounding tumors rather than by cancer cells. Hydroxamic acid-derived inhibitors of MMPs are orally bioavailable. Limited efficacy of this class of agents in clinical trials against a variety of solid tumors prompted termination of clinical trials [33,34]. MMPs are also essential to angiogenesis, preparing the tumor microenvironment for the expansion of tumor blood supply.

2-Methoxyestradiol

2-Methoxyestradiol (2ME) is a potent orally active anti-angiogenesis and anti-tumor agent of apparently minimal toxicity. Although it is an endogenous metabolite of estradiol, 2ME has not shown estrogenic activity in vitro and in vivo at doses at which estradiol and other metabolites are biologically active. 2ME is under clinical study in metastatic cancer, with and without a TKI [35].

Small Molecule Integrin Antagonists

The contributions of integrins to angiogenesis-mediated disorders have been well-described [36], as have the roles of $\alpha v\beta 3$, $\alpha v\beta 5$ [37], and $\alpha 5\beta 1$ [38] integrins in modulation of normal angiogenesis [38]. A receptor for thyroid hormone (L-thyroxine, T_4; 3,5,3′-triiodo-L-thyronine, T_3) exists on integrin $\alpha v\beta 3$ [39] and, via this site, the hormone and hormone analogs have been shown to modulate angiogenesis in the CAM and other assays. A derivative of T_4, tetraiodothyroacetic acid (tetrac), is potently anti-angiogenic at this site [6] and also has anti-cancer properties [40].

Nutraceutical-Derived Polyphenols

Phytochemicals have been shown to have anti-cancer properties, including anti-angiogenic activity. Prominent phytochemicals reported to affect angiogenic pathways include green tea polyphenols (epigallocatechin gallate, EGCG), soy bean isoflavones (genistein), and other polyphenols from natural sources [41–43].

ANTI-ANGIOGENESIS THERAPY IN HEMATOLOGIC CANCER: MULTIPLE MYELOMA

Multiple myeloma (MM) exhibits increased bone marrow neo-vascularization. Targeting host tumor-related proangiogenesis mechanisms thus became an attractive therapeutic approach to MM. Thalidomide is a glutamic acid derivative understood to have anti-angiogenic behavior in murine models. This agent has recently been found to be effective in relapsed/refractory MM. The response rate of 30–40% was associated with low-grade systemic toxicity. In addition to anti-angiogenesis, thalidomide has immunomodulatory actions and inhibits production of certain cytokines in bone marrow stroma. Studies of thalidomide-based drug combinations, for example, with dexamethasone or with conventional chemotherapy, have revealed some synergy, with up to 50–70% response rates. There is current interest in pre-clinical MM research in novel anti-angiogenic agents, including thalidomide analogs [44], inhibitors of VEGFR-2, and in end-ostatin [45]. Thalidomide and anti-VEGF (SU5416), however, have exhibited increased thrombosis risk when used in com-bination with chemotherapeutic agents [46,47]. Bortezomib has been shown to achieve improved complete response rate, progression free survival and overall survival in MM [48]. In a 3-arm randomized trial, the Spanish Myeloma Group has com-pared the combinations of bortezomib/thalidomide/dexameth-asone (VTD) versus thalidomide/dexamethasone (TD) versus vincristine, BCNU, melphalan, cyclophosphamide, prednisone/ vincristine, BCNU, doxorubicin, dexamethasone/bortezomib (VBMCP/VBAD/B) in MM. The participants were 65 years of age or younger. The primary endpoint was complete response rate postinduction and postautologous stem cell transplantation (ASCT). In this comparison, VTD was found to be a highly ef-fective induction regimen prior to ASCT [49]. See Chapter 3 for a detailed discussion of anti-angiogenesis in MM.

ANTI-COAGULANTS AND ANGIOGENESIS

A hypercoaguable state exists in many cancer patients, with risks of recurrent thrombosis attributable to the effects of cancer cells and chemotherapy on the coagulation cascade [30]. Significant increases in thrombin generation and endothelial cell perturba-tion were found to be present in a treatment cycle-dependent manner when angiogenesis inhibitors and chemotherapeutic agent therapy were combined in cancer patients [46,47]. The risk of thromboembolic events apparently related to an SU5416 and chemotherapeutic agent combination has discouraged further studies of this regimen [47]. These results and the increased risk of deep venous thrombosis (DVT) in MM patients receiving thalidomide and chemotherapeutic agents [48] prompted addition of an anti-coagulant, such as heparin or low molecular weight heparin (LMWH) in such patients. Interestingly, unfractionated heparin (UFH) or LMWH have been shown to inhibit tumor growth and metastasis. A clinically relevant survival effect of LMWH, as compared to UFH, has been shown in cancer patients with DVT. Efficacy of LMWH and its in vivo releasable tissue factor pathway inhibitor on the regulation of angiogenesis and tumor growth has been shown [50,51]. Various in vitro models and in vivo animal models have been used to show that heparin, steroids, and heparin/steroid combinations are effective inhibitors of angiogenesis [52,53]. Platelet-tumor cell interactions may contribute to metastasis [53], and drug interference with such interactions is therapeutically desirable.

POSSIBLE MECHANISMS OF ACQUIRED RESISTANCE TO ANTI-ANGIOGENIC DRUGS

It is now apparent that resistance can develop to the various types of angiogenesis inhibitors. Resistance to an agent can be based on angiogenesis or on the induction in tumor cells of apoptosis when anti-angiogenic drugs have this action. Resistance occurs even in the setting of certain primary inhibitors of angiogenesis, especially when these agents are used clinically as monotherapies [54]. Primary inhibitors are agents that directly interact with proangiogenic factors, rather than via signal transduction pathways.

There are a number of mechanisms underlying acquired resistance. First, there is redundancy of proangiogenic growth factors that may become apparent when a single drug is used to target a single vascular growth factor or its relevant receptor tyrosine kinase on endothelial cells. Second, high local concentrations of proangiogenic factors produced by cancer cells in a prosurvival mode may stoichiometrically defeat an anti-angiogenic agent and also express defensive anti-apoptotic effects. Third, transient epigenetic upregulation may occur of anti-apoptotic factors in tumor cells or endothelial cells. Thus, control of vascular supply in tumor beds appears most likely to be achieved with combinations of anti-angiogenic agents [2,54].

STANDARD CHEMOTHERAPY VERSUS ANGIOGENESIS INHIBITORS

Angiogenesis inhibitors target dividing endothelial cells rather than tumor cells. Such targeting reduces the likelihood of side effects on the skin, gastrointestinal tract, or kidney. It also reduces the risk of bone marrow toxicity in solid tumor management. Anti-angiogenic drugs may not kill tumor cells, but if vascular supply to the tumor is limited, these drugs may stabilize the cancer for an indefinite period of time. Therapeutic endpoints in this context may not be tumor shrinkage, but may be improved survival or delayed tumor progression.

Drug resistance manifested by tumors that occurs with standard cancer chemotherapy agents is common. It reflects primarily the genetic instability of cancer cells, permitting mutations that favor drug resistance.

ANTI-ANGIOGENESIS AGENTS AND THROMBOSIS

Anti-angiogenesis agents may induce endothelial cell dysfunction. The nature of such dysfunction is variable, but includes events that are associated with increased incidence of thrombosis [45–47,55].

DIAGNOSTIC IMAGING OF ANGIOGENESIS

The burgeoning interest in anti-angiogenesis strategies has highlighted a need for improved, noninvasive, quantitative techniques to serially define the anatomy and function of tumor vasculature and of peripheral and coronary vessels. These might include tumor-specific magnetic resonance and nuclear perfusion imaging of angiogenesis. Circulating biomarkers might also measure disease prognosis and treatment effectiveness [56].

microRNA AND ANGIOGENESIS MODULATION

Patterns of expression of microRNA (miRNA) have been defined in a variety of human diseases in which vascular changes are critical, for example, cardiovascular disease and cancer [57]. Pro- and anti-angiogenic strategies are possible with miRNAs because one miRNA may regulate endothelial functions by targeting multiple transcription pathways that either stimulate or inhibit blood vessel formation. Nanotechnology and targeted delivery of miRNAs or anti-miRNAs enable tumor-specific endothelial cell uptake of these agents [58]. Anti-sense technologies and RNA interference strategies provide additional information relevant to miRNA therapeutics. Serious adverse consequences of miRNA-based therapy may occur away from the target [59,60].

REFERENCES

[1] National Cancer Institute. Angiogenesis inhibitors. Available from: http://www.cancer.gov/about-cancer/treatment/types/immunotherapy/angiogenesis-inhibitors-fact-sheet

[2] Mousa SA, editor. Angiogenesis Inhibitors and Stimulators: Potential Therapeutic Implications. 1st ed. Georgetown: Eurekah.com/Landes Bioscience; 2000. p. 1–12.

[3] Pavlakovic H, Havers W, Schweigerer L. Multiple angiogenesis stimulators in a single malignancy: implications for anti-angiogenic tumour therapy. Angiogenesis 2001;4(4):259–62.

[4] Ranieri G, Gasparini G. Angiogenesis and angiogenesis inhibitors: a new potential anticancer therapeutic strategy. Curr Drug Targets Immune Endocr Metabol Disord 2001;1(3):241–53.

[5] Carmeliet P, Jain RK. Molecular mechanisms and clinical applications of angiogenesis. Nature 2011;473(7347):298–307.

[6] Mousa SA, Lin HY, Tang HY, Hercbergs A, Luidens MK, Davis PJ. Modulation of angiogenesis by thyroid hormone and hormone analogues: implications for cancer management. Angiogenesis 2014;17(3):463–9.

[7] Ali SH, O'Donnell AL, Balu D, Pohl MB, Seyler MJ, Mohamed S, Mousa S, Dandona P. Estrogen receptor-α in the inhibition of cancer growth and angiogenesis. Cancer Res 2000;60(24):7094–8.

[8] Kerbel RS. Tumor angiogenesis. N Engl J Med 2008;358(19):2039–49.

[9] Denekamp J. Limited role of vasculature-mediated injury in tumor response to radiotherapy. J Natl Cancer Inst 1993;85(12):935–7.

[10] Folkman J. Tumor angiogenesis: therapeutic implications. N Engl J Med 1971;285(21):1182–6.

[11] Chamberlain MC. Bevacizumab for the treatment of recurrent glioblastoma. Clin Med Insights Oncol 2011;5:117–29.

[12] Bottsford-Miller JN, Coleman RL, Sood AK. Resistance and escape from antiangiogenesis therapy: clinical implications and future strategies. J Clin Oncol 2012;30(32):4026–34.

[13] Kurozumi K, Ichikawa T, Onishi M, Fujii K, Date I. Cilengitide treatment for malignant glioma: current status and future direction. Neurol Med Chir (Tokyo) 2012;52(8):539–47.

[14] Scaringi C, Minniti G, Caporello P, Enrici RM. Integrin inhibitor cilengitide for the treatment of glioblastoma: a brief overview of current clinical results. Anticancer Res 2012;32(10):4213–23.

[15] Nabors LB, Fink KL, Mikkelsen T, Grujicic D, Tarnawski R, Nam DH, Mazurkiewicz M, Salacz M, Ashby L, Zagonel V, Depenni R, Perry JR, Hicking C, Picard M, Hegi ME, Lhermitte B, Reardon DA. Two cilengitide regimens in combination with standard treatment for patients with newly diagnosed glioblastoma and unmethylated *MGMT* gene promoter: results of the open-label, controlled, randomized phase II CORE study. Neuro Oncol 2015;17(5):708–17.

[16] Su J, Cai M, Li W, Hou B, He H, Ling C, Huang T, Liu H, Guo Y. Molecularly targeted drugs plus radiotherapy and temozolomide treatment for newly diagnosed glioblastoma: a meta-analysis and systematic review. Oncol Res 2016;24(2):117–28.

[17] Alva A, Slovin S, Daignault S, Carducci M, Dipaola R, Pienta K, Agus D, Cooney K, Chen A, Smith DC, Hussain M. Phase II study of cilengitide (EMD 121974, NSC 707544) in patients with non-metastatic castration resistant prostate cancer, NCI-6735. A study by the DOD/PCF prostate cancer clinical trials consortium. Invest New Drugs 2012;30(2):749–57.

[18] Davis PJ, Davis FB, Mousa SA, Luidens MK, Lin HY. Membrane receptor for thyroid hormone: physiologic and pharmacologic implications. Annu Rev Pharmacol Toxicol 2011;51:99–115.

[19] Davis PJ, Glinsky GV, Lin HY, Leith JT, Hercbergs A, Tang HY, Ashur-Fabian O, Incerpi S, Mousa SA. Cancer cell gene expression modulated

from plasma membrane integrin αvβ3 by thyroid hormone and nanoparticulate tetrac. Front Endocrinol (Lausanne) 2014;5:240.

[20] Lin HY, Sun M, Lin C, Tang HY, London D, Shih A, Davis FB, Davis PJ. Androgen-induced human breast cancer cell proliferation is mediated by discrete mechanisms in estrogen receptor-α-positive and -negative breast cancer cells. J Steroid Biochem Mol Biol 2009;113(3–5):182–8.

[21] Lin HY, Lansing L, Merillon JM, Davis FB, Tang HY, Shih A, Vitrac X, Krisa S, Keating T, Cao HJ, Bergh J, Quackenbush S, Davis PJ. Integrin αVβ3 contains a receptor site for resveratrol. FASEB J 2006;20(10): 1742–4.

[22] Belcik JT, Qi Y, Kaufmann BA, Xie A, Bullens S, Morgan TK, Bagby SP, Kolumam G, Kowalski J, Oyer JA, Bunting S, Lindner JR. Cardiovascular and systemic microvascular effects of anti-vascular endothelial growth factor therapy for cancer. J Am Coll Cardiol 2012;60(7): 618–25.

[23] Chen HX, Cleck JN. Adverse effects of anticancer agents that target the VEGF pathway. Nat Rev Clin Oncol 2009;6(8):465–77.

[24] Rapisarda A, Melillo G. Overcoming disappointing results with antiangiogenic therapy by targeting hypoxia. Nat Rev Clin Oncol 2012;9(7): 378–90.

[25] Bergers G, Hanahan D. Modes of resistance to anti-angiogenic therapy. Nat Rev Cancer 2008;8(8):592–603.

[26] Small AC, Oh WK. Bevacizumab treatment of prostate cancer. Expert Opin Biol Ther 2012;12(9):1241–9.

[27] de Groot JF, Lamborn KR, Chang SM, Gilbert MR, Cloughesy TF, Aldape K, Yao J, Jackson EF, Lieberman F, Robins HI, Mehta MP, Lassman AB, Deangelis LM, Yung WK, Chen A, Prados MD, Wen PY. Phase II study of aflibercept in recurrent malignant glioma: a North American Brain Tumor Consortium study. J Clin Oncol 2011;29(19):2689–95.

[28] Mitchell P. A systematic review of the efficacy and safety outcomes of anti-VEGF agents used for treating neovascular age-related macular degeneration: comparison of ranibizumab and bevacizumab. Curr Med Res Opin 2011;27(7):1465–75.

[29] Chong V. Biological, preclinical and clinical characteristics of inhibitors of vascular endothelial growth factors. Ophthalmologica 2012;227 (Suppl. 1):2–10.

[30] Colman RW, Jameson BA, Lin Y, Johnson D, Mousa SA. Domain 5 of high molecular weight kininogen (kininostatin) down-regulates endothelial cell proliferation and migration and inhibits angiogenesis. Blood 2000;95(2):543–50.

[31] Shahan T, Grant D, Tootell M, Ziaie Z, Ohno N, Mousa S, Mohamad S, Delisser H, Kefalides N. Oncothanin, a peptide from the α3 chain of type IV collagen, modifies endothelial cell function and inhibits angiogenesis. Connect Tissue Res 2004;45(3):151–63.

[32] Sudhakar A, Boosani CS. Inhibition of tumor angiogenesis by tumstatin: insights into signaling mechanisms and implications in cancer regression. Pharm Res 2008;25(12):2731–9.

[33] Moore MJ, Hamm J, Dancey J, Eisenberg PD, Dagenais M, Fields A, Hagan K, Greenberg B, Colwell B, Zee B, Tu D, Ottaway J, Humphrey R, Seymour L. Comparison of gemcitabine versus the matrix metallopro-teinase inhibitor BAY 12-9566 in patients with advanced or metastatic adenocarcinoma of the pancreas: a phase III trial of the National Cancer Institute of Canada Clinical Trials Group. J Clin Oncol 2003;21(17): 3296–302.

[34] Rudek MA, Figg WD, Dyer V, Dahut W, Turner ML, Steinberg SM, Liewehr DJ, Kohler DR, Pluda JM, Reed E. Phase I clinical trial of oral COL-3, a matrix metalloproteinase inhibitor, in patients with refractory metastatic cancer. J Clin Oncol 2001;19(2):584–92.

[35] Bruce JY, Eickhoff J, Pili R, Logan T, Carducci M, Arnott J, Treston A, Wilding G, Liu G. A phase II study of 2-methoxyestradiol nanocrystal colloidal dispersion alone and in combination with sunitinib malate in pa-tients with metastatic renal cell carcinoma progressing on sunitinib malate. Invest New Drugs 2012;30(2):794–802.

[36] Mousa SA. IBC's Sixth Annual Conference on Angiogenesis: novel thera-peutic developments. Expert Opin Investig Drugs 2001;10(2):387–91.

[37] Van Waes C, Enamorado-Ayala I, Hecht D, Sulica L, Chen Z, Batt DG, Mousa S. Effects of the novel alphav integrin antagonist SM256 and cis-platinum on growth of murine squamous cell carcinoma PAM LY8. Int J Oncol 2000;16(6):1189–95.

[38] Kim S, Bell K, Mousa SA, Varner JA. Regulation of angiogenesis in vivo by ligation of integrin α5β1 with the central cell-binding domain of fibronectin. Am J Pathol 2000;156(4):1345–62.

[39] Davis PJ, Davis FB, Mousa SA, Luidens MK, Lin HY. Membrane recep-tor for thyroid hormone: physiologic and pharmacologic implications. Annu Rev Pharmacol Toxicol 2011;51:99–115.

[40] Davis PJ, Goglia F, Leonard JL. Nongenomic actions of thyroid hormone. Nat Rev Endocrinol 2016;12(2):111–21.

[41] Siddiqui IA, Adhami VM, Bharali DJ, Hafeez BB, Asim M, Khwaja SI, Ahmad N, Cui H, Mousa SA, Mukhtar H. Introducing nanochemopre-vention as a novel approach for cancer control: proof of principle with

green tea polyphenol epigallocatechin-3-gallate. Cancer Res 2009;69(5): 1712–6.

[42] Nguyen MM, Ahmann FR, Nagle RB, Hsu CH, Tangrea JA, Parnes HL, Sokoloff MH, Gretzer MB, Chow HH. Randomized, double-blind, placebo-controlled trial of polyphenon E in prostate cancer patients before prostatectomy: evaluation of potential chemopreventive activities. Cancer Prev Res (Phila) 2012;5(2):290–8.

[43] Kanai M, Yoshimura K, Asada M, Imaizumi A, Suzuki C, Matsumoto S, Nishimura T, Mori Y, Masui T, Kawaguchi Y, Yanagihara K, Yazumi S, Chiba T, Guha S, Aggarwal BB. A phase I/II study of gemcitabine-based chemotherapy plus curcumin for patients with gemcitabine-resistant pancreatic cancer. Cancer Chemother Pharmacol 2011;68(1):157–64.

[44] Brower V. Lenalidomide maintenance for multiple myeloma. Lancet Oncol 2012;13(6):e238.

[45] Tosi P, Tura S. Antiangiogenic therapy in multiple myeloma. Acta Haematol 2001;106(4):208–13.

[46] Bennett CL, Schumock GT, Desai AA, Kwaan HC, Raisch DW, Newlin R, Stadler W. Thalidomide-associated deep vein thrombosis and pulmonary embolism. Am J Med 2002;113(7):603–6.

[47] Kuenen BC, Rosen L, Smit EF, Parson MR, Levi M, Ruijter R, Huisman H, Kedde MA, Noordhuis P, van der Vijgh WJ, Peters GJ, Cropp GF, Scigalla P, Hoekman K, Pinedo HM, Giaccone G. Dose-finding and pharmacokinetic study of cisplatin, gemcitabine, and SU5416 in patients with solid tumors. J Clin Oncol 2002;20(6):1657–67.

[48] Sonneveld P, Schmidt-Wolf IG, van der Holt B, El Jarari L, Bertsch U, Salwender H, Zweegman S, Vellenga E, Broyl A, Blau IW, Weisel KC, Wittebol S, Bos GM, Stevens-Kroef M, Scheid C, Pfreundschuh M, Hose D, Jauch A, van der Velde H, Raymakers R, Schaafsma MR, Kersten MJ, van Marwijk-Kooy M, Duehrsen U, Lindemann W, Wijermans PW, Lokhorst HM, Goldschmidt HM. Bortezomib induction and maintenance treatment in patients with newly diagnosed multiple myeloma: results of the randomized phase III HOVON-65/GMMG-HD4 trial. J Clin Oncol 2012;30(24):2946–55.

[49] Rosinol L, Oriol A, Teruel AI, Hernandez D, Lopez-Jimenez J, de la Rubia J, Granell M, Besalduch J, Palomera L, Gonzalez Y, Etxebeste MA, Diaz-Mediavilla J, Hernandez MT, de Arriba F, Gutierrez NC, Martin-Ramos ML, Cibeira MT, Mateos MV, Martinez J, Alegre A, Lahuerta JJ, San Miguel J, Blade J. Programa para el Estudio y la Terapeutica de las Hemopatias Malignas/Grupo Espanol de Mieloma g. Superiority of bortezomib, thalidomide, and dexamethasone (VTD) as induction pretransplantation

therapy in multiple myeloma: a randomized phase 3 PETHEMA/GEM study. Blood 2012;120(8):1589–96.

[50] Mousa SA. Anticoagulants in thrombosis and cancer: the missing link. Semin Thromb Hemost 2002;28(1):45–52.

[51] Mousa SA, Mohamed S. Anti-angiogenic mechanisms and efficacy of the low molecular weight heparin, tinzaparin: anti-cancer efficacy. Oncol Rep 2004;12(4):683–8.

[52] Jung SP, Siegrist B, Wade MR, Anthony CT, Woltering EA. Inhibition of human angiogenesis with heparin and hydrocortisone. Angiogenesis 2001;4(3):175–86.

[53] McCarty OJT, Mousa SA, Bray PF, Konstantopoulos K. Immobilized platelets support human colon carcinoma cell tethering, rolling, and firm adhesion under dynamic flow conditions. Blood 2000;96(5):1789–97.

[54] Kerbel RS, Yu J, Tran J, Man S, Viloria-Petit A, Klement G, Coomber BL, Rak J. Possible mechanisms of acquired resistance to anti-angiogenic drugs: implications for the use of combination therapy approaches. Cancer Metastasis Rev 2001;20(1–2):79–86.

[55] Kaushal V, Kohli M, Zangari M, Fink L, Mehta P. Endothelial dysfunction in antiangiogenesis-associated thrombosis. J Clin Oncol 2002;20(13):3042.

[56] Chen Z, Malhotra PS, Thomas GR, Ondrey FG, Duffey DC, Smith CW, Enamorado I, Yeh NT, Kroog GS, Rudy S, McCullagh L, Mousa S, Quezado M, Herscher LL, Van Waes C. Expression of proinflammatory and proangiogenic cytokines in patients with head and neck cancer. Clin Cancer Res 1999;5(6):1369–79.

[57] Liu N, Olson EN. MicroRNA regulatory networks in cardiovascular development. Dev Cell 2010;18(4):510–25.

[58] Murphy EA, Majeti BK, Barnes LA, Makale M, Weis SM, Lutu-Fuga K, Wrasidlo W, Cheresh DA. Nanoparticle-mediated drug delivery to tumor vasculature suppresses metastasis. Proc Natl Acad Sci USA 2008;105(27):9343–8.

[59] Heusschen R, van Gink M, Griffioen AW, Thijssen VL. MicroRNAs in the tumor endothelium: novel controls on the angioregulatory switchboard. Biochim Biophys Acta 2010;1805(1):87–96.

[60] Rayner KJ, Suarez Y, Davalos A, Parathath S, Fitzgerald ML, Tamehiro N, Fisher EA, Moore KJ, Fernandez-Hernando C. MiR-33 contributes to the regulation of cholesterol homeostasis. Science 2010;328(5985):1570–3.

CHAPTER 2

Models for Assessing Anti-Angiogenesis Agents: Appraisal of Current Techniques

Shaker A. Mousa, Murat Yalcin and Paul J. Davis

Contents

The development of anti- and proangiogenic pharmaceuticals and investigation of mechanisms of action of naturally occurring factors that regulate new blood vessel formation require in vitro and in vivo assay systems. A number of these are listed in Table 2.1. Ideal assays are quantitative and reproducible, rapid, cost effective, and relevant to angiogenesis in clinical practice. We define "relevance" here to mean that the angiogenic process that is captured: (1) responds to human vascular growth factors and small molecules that have angiogenic properties and (2) depends upon structural proteins, for example, integrins, of the plasma membrane

Table 2.1 Angiogenesis models

In vitro models	In vivo models
Cultured EC on different substratum: Matrigel Collagen/fibronectin Laminin Fibrin or gelatin Sprouting from aortic rings	Matrigel in mice Chick chorioallantoic membrane-CAM assay Rabbit cornea Hypoxia/ischemia–induced retinal/iris NV in rats, mice, primates Laser-induced choroidal NV Human skin/human tumor transplanted on SCID mice Tumor metastatic models in mice

CAM, Chorioallantoic membrane; EC, endothelial cell; NV, neovascularization.
Source: With permission of Springer: Mousa SA, Davis PJ. Angiogenesis Modulations in Health and Disease, Chapter 1 Angiogenesis Assays: An Appraisal of Current Techniques, 2013, p. 1–12.

of endothelial cells in the assay system that are very comparable to those in human cells. Certain angiogenesis assays can incorporate tumor cells and permit these cells to regulate the ongoing, intrinsic blood vessel formation of the assay; such assays are clearly attractive for studies of cancer-associated angiogenesis. The chick chorioallantoic membrane (CAM) model involves angiogenesis at the time of very early embryogenesis, but away from the embryo, and is immune-tolerant of tumor cells from another species. Tumors implanted in the CAM may also grow spherically, mimicking clinical cancer growth and reproducing the oxygen differential across clinical tumor diameter.

An initial question in choice of a blood vessel formation assay is whether the studies are to be of vasculogenesis, that is, related to the developmental process, or of angiogenesis; the latter is not linked to development. Angiogenesis will involve differentiation of angioblasts into endothelial cells before vessel sprouting occurs. In the in vivo methods presented later, the CAM assay examines *angiogenesis*, while the zebrafish embryo assay features *vasculogenesis*. The zebrafish model however, does include identifiable vessels participating in angiogenesis.

A number of reviews are available of angiogenesis assays [1–5] and the history of such assays [6]. The features of a select group of widely applied angiogenesis assays are reviewed here. These systems can be readily reproduced in the laboratory. All of these models bear the risk of failure to predict clinical response to angiogenesis-directed pharmaceuticals because of the phylogenetic gulf that exists between (preclinical) animal models and human subjects.

IN VIVO ASSAYS
Chick Chorioallantoic Membrane

Introduced by Folkman et al., in 1974 [7], the CAM assay is the most widely used in vivo angiogenesis assay [8–10]. It offers a sound vascular structure in which to study tumor growth, angiogenic and anti-angiogenic molecules. The conventional application involves the cutting of a resealable small window in the shell of an egg containing a developing embryo and then insertion of test substance(s) on filter discs and/or a xenograft through the shell window. Effects on new blood vessel generation are monitored for 3 or more days. The shell window is sealed between manipulations because the CAM is sensitive to oxygen tension. Scoring of angiogenesis is: (1) by number of vessels and vessel branch points, (2) by microscope visualization of the membrane about the site of the test substance filter disc or xenograft, (3) both approaches, and (4) by application of a software template to images of the membrane (Fig. 2.1; [11]). The software measurement may be automated. An alternative system involves explanting the embryo and CAM to a Petri dish without the shell and then quantitating angiogenesis.

Readily reproducible and inexpensive, the CAM model also is ideal for fast, large-scale screening of test drugs, antibodies, vasoactive peptides, or growth factors [12]. The chorioallantoic membrane may be sampled for biochemical analysis—for example, signal transducing enzyme activities, vascular growth factor assays—as well as for histology and histopathology. A critical feature of the CAM assay is its dependence upon integrin $\alpha v\beta 3$ expressed in the plasma

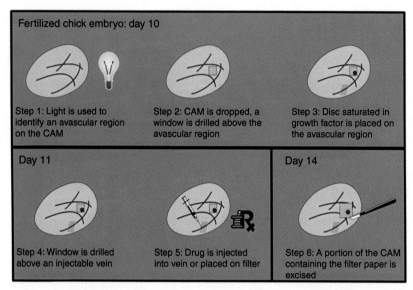

Figure 2.1 *Stepwise protocol for growth factor-induced angiogenesis in the chick chorioallantoic membrane (CAM) model. (With permission of Springer: Mousa SA, Davis PJ. Angiogenesis Modulations in Health and Disease, Chapter 1 Angiogenesis Assays: An Appraisal of Current Techniques, 2013, p. 1–12).*

membrane of the rapidly dividing chick endothelial cell. This feature of the system has enabled identification of small molecule receptor sites on the integrin, including the receptor for thyroid hormone [13–15]. Mammalian vascular growth factors, such as vascular endothelial growth factor (VEGF) or basic fibroblast growth factor (bFGF, FGF2), are easily assayed in the CAM (Fig. 2.2). Evaluation of anti-angiogenic agents is also conventionally done in this model (Fig. 2.3). Tumor xenografts may invade the embryo in each fertilized (CAM) egg and this permits evaluation of tumor aggressiveness in the presence or absence of test materials administered via the filter discs. The basal rate of angiogenesis is generous in the CAM, and pharmaceuticals or other agents with low-potency angiogenic activity may not be suitable for evaluation in this system. The CAM provides information about the timing of onset of effects of pro- or anti-angiogenic test substances, but possible insights into decay pharmacokinetics may be obtained only with the removal of the

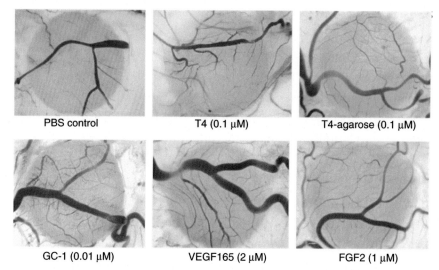

Figure 2.2 *Representative images of effects of inducers of angiogenesis in the CAM model.* T4, T4-agarose, and GC-1 are the thyroid hormone-based proangiogenic compounds (13–15). *(With permission of Springer: Mousa SA, Davis PJ. Angiogenesis Modulations in Health and Disease, Chapter 1 Angiogenesis Assays: An Appraisal of Current Techniques, 2013, p. 1–12).*

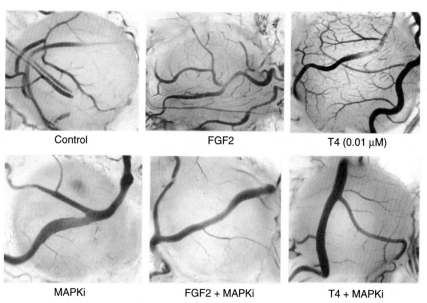

Figure 2.3 *Representative images for examining the potential mechanisms of proangiogenesis mediators in the CAM model.* The MAPK inhibitor (MAPKi) in these studies was PD98059 [16]. *(With permission of Springer: Mousa SA, Davis PJ. Angiogenesis Modulations in Health and Disease, Chapter 1 Angiogenesis Assays: An Appraisal of Current Techniques, 2013, p. 1–12).*

filter discs containing the test substances from the CAM and assaying residual content. The CAM is immune-tolerant, but occasional inflammatory responses occur near the xenografts. On the other hand, the capacity of the membrane to express inflammation may be useful in studies involving the inflammatory response.

Zebrafish

A tropical freshwater fish, the zebrafish generates embryos that are easily cultivated in the laboratory. A single mating results in the development of hundreds of embryos that are yolk sac-dependent and develop outside the mother. Because the embryos are optically clear, their organ development and emergence of blood vessels can be readily seen by microscope [17]. Confocal microscopy and angiography have also been used to monitor angiogenesis. Transgenic zebrafish that express green fluorescent protein (GFP) variants are now available and have improved vessel visualization. Another transgenic model features erythrocytes labeled with a second fluorescent dye that permits blood flow to be monitored concomitantly with GFP-profiled blood vessel formation. The small size and the optical clarity of the zebrafish embryo in combination with the advancements in imaging technologies cleared the way for the zebrafish to be an important in vivo model for testing angiogenic and anti-angiogenic molecules [18].

Because the zebrafish model is wholly focused on embryo development, distinction between vasculogenesis and angiogenesis is essential in studies of pharmacologic agents or growth factors in this assay. This distinction is made anatomically. That is, intersegment blood vessels are seen to reflect *angiogenesis* in which endothelial cells develop from primordial vessel cells prior to sprouting. In contrast, the dorsal aorta is a component of embryonic *vasculogenesis* from which this differentiation is absent. The zebrafish model may be subjected to specific gene knockdowns with small interfering RNAs (siRNAs) that enable assessment of function of genes of interest.

How homologous fish circulation and fish angiogenesis are to human cancer-associated angiogenesis is not clear. The route of administration for testing of pharmaceuticals or of bioproducts may be complex in this model. As an example, proteins must be administered via the yolk sac. In contrast, however, small lipophilic compounds can be added to the water in which the fish reside and will be absorbed by the embryos.

Subcutaneous and Orthotopic Xenografts

For studies of tumor biology and relevant angiogenesis, it is attractive to study orthotopic tumor implants (xenografts) in which the local microenvironment resembles that in human cancers [3]. Subcutaneous tumor implants are less desirable from the standpoint of modeling the condition in patients, but these are a technically convenient option for the studying of dose escalation of single drugs and for comparing effects of multiple agents. The blood vessel supply about tumor xenografts is generous. This permits histologic and biochemical analysis. In addition, a simplified index of vascularity, for example, tumor hemoglobin content, is straightforward in subcutaneous xenografts, and the technical expertise needed for many types of orthotopic insertion is avoided. Two weeks is sufficient for the establishment of most xenografts, after which drug or factor testing is initiated and continues for several weeks. Subcutaneous xenograft volumes may be estimated daily by calipers, and subsets of animals can be sacrificed periodically during treatment in order to obtain histology and biochemical information that is needed. The few weeks required for each drug or factor study yields substantial amounts of information and is consistent with needs to secure data about multiple drugs, drug dosages, or combinations of drugs (Fig. 2.3). From the standpoints of angiogenesis and tumor cell biology, the subcutaneous xenograft model is a useful screening option in studies of angiogenesis.

Tumor measurements length, width, and height are feasible when papable tumors are present and this usually occurs within 7 days after subcutaneous tumor cell inoculation. However, tumor size is a function of cancer cell type. Quantitation of angiogenesis in xenografts is feasible with CD31 immunostaining, with other endothelial cell markers or by spectrophotometric estimation of hemoglobin content using Drabkin's reagent.

Orthotopic human tumor implants in the nude mouse closely mimic the local microenvironmental conditions of the primary clinical tumor. Tumor behaviors and the activity of the associated vasculature reflect the interaction of local host factors with the intrinsic qualities of the cancer cells [19]. Interstitial pressure generation in orthotopic tumors is likely to be quite different from that achieved with subcutaneous implantation. Increased interstitial pressure of course restricts access of systemically administered drugs, including angiogenesis-relevant agents, to tumor cells. In addition, certain qualities of blood vessels are distinctive at the orthotopic site. Among such qualities are microvessel density, blood vessel permeability, and blood vessel cell gene expression [20]. Transcriptional differences among implantation sites, depending on the tumor cell type, have involved tumor genes for *FGF2* (*bFGF*), for *VEGF*, and VEGF receptors and, importantly, for genes involved in the development of multidrug resistance and in supporting inflammation [3].

The nude mouse is small and this enables serial nonradioisotopic fluorescence IVIS imaging (in vivo imaging system) of orthotopic cancer implants (Fig. 2.4; [21]), yielding information about tumor volumes that is more accurate than noninvasive volume estimates of subcutaneous xenografts. IVIS scans also distinguish viable cells from dead cells in tumor mass and may be used to measure other qualities of the cells in the scanned xenograft.

Matrigel Plug Assay

Matrigel or collagen or fibrin matrices have been described in which endothelial cell differentiation may be estimated in response to vascular growth factors, to other proangiogenic factors, and to anti-angiogenic agents. These matrices have been used in both in vitro and in vivo models. Endothelial cell differentiation is vessel sprouting or microtubule formation in these models, and which manifestation is observed depends on the composition of the matrix. In Matrigel it is tubule formation that results. Matrigel

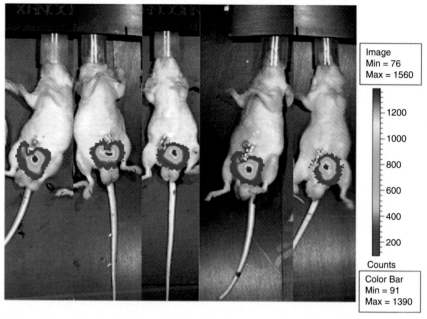

Figure 2.4 *Representative IVIS images taken 1 week after orthotopic implantation of prostate cancer cells (PC3-Luc) in male nude mice.* Loss of cell viability is tracked by bioluminescent color change [red (actively dividing cells) to blue]. *(With permission of Springer: Mousa SA, Davis PJ. Angiogenesis Modulations in Health and Disease, Chapter 1 Angiogenesis Assays: An Appraisal of Current Techniques, 2013, p. 1–12).*

plugs to which a vascular growth factor has been added result in quantifiable host blood vessel-based angiogenesis in the plug. Matrigel is made up of mouse sarcoma extracellular matrix proteins and basement membrane proteins. A solid gel at 37°C, Matrigel is a liquid at 4°C. It also contains murine vascular growth factors imbedded in the extracellular matrix of mouse sarcoma. Matrigel is also available in a form lacking some of the mouse proangiogenic factors associated with the sarcoma.

We have used an in vivo protocol [11,22] in which host vascularization of plugs develops over 7–14 days. In this system, one or several subcutaneous injections per mouse contain standard volumes of Matrigel, for example, 100 μL, to which is added a vascular growth factor. Then, an anti-angiogenesis drug or factor is systemically administered. Hemoglobin content of standard volumes of harvested aliquots of plugs is an easily measured index of angiogenesis, but histologic examination also provides semiquantitative estimates of angiogenesis. Knowledge of the pharmacokinetics of the test substance(s) is required to use this approach. Assay duration is similar to that of xenograft models.

IN VITRO ASSAYS
Aortic Ring Assay

Standardized in the mouse, this assay involves harvest of the thoracic aorta, excision of the adventitia and then the serial cutting of rings 1 mm in length that are implanted in collagen gels [23,24]. Seven days of ring culture in serum-free medium results in outgrowth of new vessels that can be examined by microscopy and by immunohistochemical staining, then compared with rings exposed to drug or growth factor. This assay can be carried out in transgenic animals in which factors that contribute to angiogenesis have been manipulated. The rat aorta has also been used and yields a greater number of rings. This is a technically difficult assay; incomplete excision of the adventitia and strain and age of mouse may influence vessel outgrowth [1].

Sprouting Assay

Vessel sprouting can be induced by vascular growth factors in cultures of endothelial cells. In vitro methods have been developed that exploit sprouting, which can be induced in confluent monolayers of endothelial cells on fibrin gels. Alternatively, the cells can be grown to confluence on microbeads; these are suspended in fibrin gel and exposed to test substances. Quantitation of sprouting is by microscopy in the standard assay. When the microbead assay is used, sprouting from a bead is reflected in measurements of vessel length or the numbers of vessels/bead.

We have used human dermal microvascular endothelial cells (HDMECs) grown to confluence over several days on gelatin-coated Cytodex-3 beads, which are exposed to normal human serum and then placed in fibrin that undergoes polymerization [25]. Anti- or proangiogenic agents may then be tested in the system within 48 h. In this model we have stimulated angiogenesis with FGF2 or VEGF and then have demonstrated the anti-angiogenic activity of a thyroid hormone derivative, tetraiodothyroacetic acid (tetrac) [11], whose receptor site is on integrin $\alpha v \beta 3$ [13].

Tube Formation Assay

Angiogenesis requires nascent blood vessel tube formation from endothelial cells [26,27]. Tubes can be induced in plate-cultured endothelial cells exposed to extracellular matrix components, such as those found in Matrigel. Human umbilical vein endothelial cells (HUVECs) or HDMECs are plated on Matrigel for this assay. Quantitation of anti-angiogenic or proangiogenic activity of substances assayed involves analysis of photographs of plate wells, estimating length and area of capillary-like structures (CLS)/unit area (Fig. 2.5). The assay can be carried out in as little as 1 day.

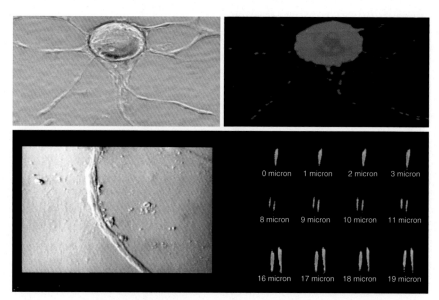

Figure 2.5 *Representative images of tube formation using three dimensional tube formation assay. (With permission of Springer: Mousa SA, Davis PJ. Angiogenesis Modulations in Health and Disease, Chapter 1 Angiogenesis Assays: An Appraisal of Current Techniques, 2013, p. 1–12).*

Contributions from murine vascular growth factors in Matrigel preparations are a source of noise in this model. The integrity of the CLS measurement must be assured in the assay by documenting the presence of lumens in the vessels, since an endothelial cell may mimic tube formation by constructing bridges or cords to adjacent cells. Fibroblasts and other cells may form networks on Matrigel [28], and cultured endothelial cells in this system must be free of contamination with fibroblasts or cancer cells that are prone to form networks when exposed to Matrigel.

THREE-DIMENSIONAL MATRIX ARRAY ULTRASOUND MOLECULAR IMAGING

Function of VEGF receptor (VEGFR)-2 can be assessed by a 3D ultrasound molecular imaging (3DUSMI) assay. A proof-of-concept study of the 3DUSMI assay predicted treatment responders versus nonresponders to anti-angiogenesis therapy for tumors implanted in a mouse model and treated with anti-VEGF. In responding tumors, the VEGFR signal decreased early after therapy, predicting treatment outcome, whereas in nonresponding tumors there was no change in VEGFR signal at any time posttreatment [29]. Further studies with various anti-angiogenesis strategies in different tumors are required to validate this model system.

COCULTURE OF HUMAN CANCER CELLS WITH HUMAN MICROVASCULAR ENDOTHELIAL CELLS

Endothelial cell sprouting and formation of capillaries has been quantitated in a 2-chamber coculture system, utilizing human lung carcinoma [30,31] or murine breast carcinoma-induced angiogenesis [32,33]. Capillaries sprout from a confluent endothelial cell monolayer after coculture with cancer cells is initiated, and this sprouting is subject to quantitation. A schematic diagram of the coculture model is shown in Fig. 2.6. There is a Transwell insert in each well, together with a polycarbonate membrane (M), 10 μm

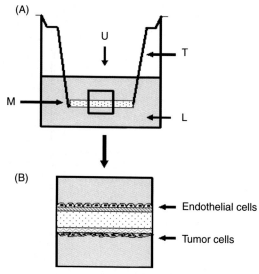

Figure 2.6 *A schematic diagram and description of the coculture model.* (A) Each well contains a Transwell insert (*T*), with a polycarbonate membrane (*M*). Insert (*T*) delineates upper chamber (*U*) from lower chamber (*L*) with the levels of media equal in both chambers. (B) Represents magnification of the separations between both chambers. *Top arrow* points to endothelial cells seeded in the upper chamber on reduced growth factor (RGF)-Matrigel-coated surface and *bottom arrow* points to cancer cells seeded on type I collagen. *(With permission of Springer: Mousa SA, Davis PJ. Angiogenesis Modulations in Health and Disease, Chapter 1 Angiogenesis Assays: An Appraisal of Current Techniques, 2013, p. 1–12).*

thick with 0.8 μm pores. The insert delineates upper chamber (U) and lower chamber (L) of the system. The amount of culture media is equal in both chambers. The upper chamber contains endothelial cells cultured on a Matrigel-coated, basement membrane–like surface and the lower chamber contains tumor cells seeded on type I collagen. Individual cell populations can be manipulated separately until the time of coculture. Test reagents can be placed in upper, lower, or both compartments. Capillary formation is evaluated by staining of endothelial cells with endothelial cell–specific CD31/PECAM antibody followed by quantification of digital images as previously described [31].

A 3D in vitro angiogenesis model using gelatin methacrylate hydrogel microwells to simulate an in vivo-like microenvironment for cocultured glioblastoma and endothelial has been used to screen various anti-angiogenesis strategies [34].

Quantitating the motility response of endothelial cell or fibroblasts to angiogenic agents under evaluation is a desirable measurement. The approach used conventionally is the Boyden chamber apparatus, in which cells migrate through a porous membrane from an upper to a lower chamber. The latter contains a biochemical cue, such as an extracellular matrix protein [35].

DISCUSSION

The ideal angiogenesis assay would be a skin window in a subhuman primate to permit direct application of angiogenesis-relevant agents and microscopy to monitor blood vessel formation that results. Alternatively, angiogenesis can be monitored after systemic administration of anti- or proangiogenesis factors. This assay does not exist. It would be valid for studies of wound-healing-related angiogenesis, but would not be useful for neovascularization associated with various tumors, where orthotopic models are best.

A complement of widely used assays has been discussed here. The usefulness of each of these has been validated and each has provided useful insights into the actions of specific pro- or antiangiogenic pharmaceuticals or to the properties of naturally occurring factors that control angiogenesis. Each model has shortcomings. It is customary for several assays to be used in the evaluation of new pharmaceutical strategies for regulation of blood vessel formation. Strategically, one should have available a cost effective, usually large-scale, screening method that enables initial estimations of dosing, of comparison of congeners, of conjoint studies with naturally occurring proangiogenic active substances and of combinations of agents. A second method should be available to confirm pro- or anti-angiogenic activity and, if the model's mechanisms are sufficiently understood, to support initial studies of the molecular basis of drug or factor action. Intact animal models are then to be exploited to validate effectiveness in ischemia-reperfusion injury, wound-healing, and disruption of oncology-related angiogenesis. Effectiveness in these systems requires quantitative and qualitative histopathology, blood vessel radiology, and high resolution in vivo imaging systems [36]. Quantitative histopathology will document numbers of small vessels and capillaries in response to interventions. Fluorescent dye options and microcomputerized tomography should be available in the imaging systems.

Elucidating the mechanisms by which angiogenesis-relevant pharmaceuticals act increasingly requires models in which specific components of angiogenesis—such as components of signal transduction systems—are deleted in target blood vessel cells by siRNAs. This approach can be applied to several of the assay systems described here and the in vitro endothelial cell-fibroblast coculture system is a particularly attractive approach in which to exploit this modification [32].

CONCLUSIONS

In this chapter, multiple in vitro and in vivo preclinical models were presented for the evaluation of angiogenesis modulator (pro- or anti-angiogenesis) agents. However, each model system has its own limitations, and the ultimate model for testing anti-angiogenesis strategies would be in a human with accelerated pathological angiogenesis, such as is the case in cancer.

REFERENCES

[1] Goodwin AM. In vitro assays of angiogenesis for assessment of angiogenic and anti-angiogenic agents. Microvasc Res 2007;74(2–3):172–83.

[2] Jensen LD, Cao R, Cao Y. In vivo angiogenesis and lymphangiogenesis models. Curr Mol Med 2009;9(8):982–91.

[3] Loi M, Di Paolo D, Becherini P, Zorzoli A, Perri P, Carosio R, Cilli M, Ribatti D, Brignole C, Pagnan G, Ponzoni M, Pastorino F. The use of the orthotopic model to validate antivascular therapies for cancer. Int J Dev Biol 2011;55(4–5):547–55.

[4] Staton CA, Reed MW, Brown NJ. A critical analysis of current in vitro and in vivo angiogenesis assays. Int J Exp Pathol 2009;90(3):195–221.

[5] Ucuzian AA, Greisler HP. In vitro models of angiogenesis. World J Surg 2007;31(4):654–63.

[6] Cimpean AM, Ribatti D, Raica M. A brief history of angiogenesis assays. Int J Dev Biol 2011;55(4–5):377–82.

[7] Auerbach R, Kubai L, Knighton D, Folkman J. A simple procedure for the long-term cultivation of chicken embryos. Dev Biol 1974;41(2):391–4.

[8] Mousa SS, Mousa SS, Mousa SA. Effect of resveratrol on angiogenesis and platelet/fibrin-accelerated tumor growth in the chick chorioallantoic membrane model. Nutr Cancer 2005;52(1):59–65.

[9] Ribatti D, Conconi MT, Nussdorfer GG. Nonclassic endogenous novel regulators of angiogenesis. Pharmacol Rev 2007;59(2):185–205.

[10] Vargas A, Zeisser-Labouebe M, Lange N, Gurny R, Delie F. The chick embryo and its chorioallantoic membrane (CAM) for the in vivo evaluation of drug delivery systems. Adv Drug Deliv Rev 2007;59(11):1162–76.

[11] Mousa SA, Bergh JJ, Dier E, Rebbaa A, O'Connor LJ, Yalcin M, Aljada A, Dyskin E, Davis FB, Lin HY, Davis PJ. Tetraiodothyroacetic acid, a small molecule integrin ligand, blocks angiogenesis induced by vascular endothelial growth factor and basic fibroblast growth factor. Angiogenesis 2008;11(2):183–90.

[12] Ribatti D. The chick embryo chorioallantoic membrane (CAM). A multifaceted experimental model. Mech Dev 2016;141:70–7.

[13] Bergh JJ, Lin HY, Lansing L, Mohamed SN, Davis FB, Mousa S, Davis PJ. Integrin αvβ3 contains a cell surface receptor site for thyroid hormone that is linked to activation of mitogen-activated protein kinase and induction of angiogenesis. Endocrinology 2005;146(7):2864–71.

[14] Davis PJ, Davis FB, Mousa SA, Luidens MK, Lin HY. Membrane receptor for thyroid hormone: physiologic and pharmacologic implications. Annu Rev Pharmacol Toxicol 2011;51:99–115.

[15] Davis PJ, Davis FB, Mousa SA. Thyroid hormone-induced angiogenesis. Curr Cardiol Rev 2009;5(1):12–6.

[16] Lin HY, Davis FB, Gordinier JK, Martino LJ, Davis PJ. Thyroid hormone induces activation of mitogen-activated protein kinase in cultured cells. Am J Physiol 1999;276(5 Pt. 1):C1014–24.

[17] Tobia C, De Sena G, Presta M. Zebrafish embryo, a tool to study tumor angiogenesis. Int J Dev Biol 2011;55(4–5):505–9.

[18] Schuermann A, Helker CS, Herzog W. Angiogenesis in zebrafish. Semin Cell Dev Biol 2014;31:106–14.

[19] Talmadge JE, Donkor M, Scholar E. Inflammatory cell infiltration of tumors: Jekyll or Hyde. Cancer Metastasis Rev 2007;26(3–4):373–400.

[20] Langenkamp E, Molema G. Microvascular endothelial cell heterogeneity: general concepts and pharmacological consequences for anti-angiogenic therapy of cancer. Cell Tissue Res 2009;335(1):205–22.

[21] Yalcin M, Lin HY, Sudha T, Bharali DJ, Meng R, Tang HY, Davis FB, Stain SC, Davis PJ, Mousa SA. Response of human pancreatic cancer cell xenografts to tetraiodothyroacetic acid nanoparticles. Horm Cancer 2013;4(3):176–85.

[22] Powell JA, Mohamed SN, Kerr JS, Mousa SA. Antiangiogenesis efficacy of nitric oxide donors. J Cell Biochem 2000;80(1):104–14.

[23] Nicosia RF, Ottinetti A. Modulation of microvascular growth and morphogenesis by reconstituted basement membrane gel in three-dimensional cultures of rat aorta: a comparative study of angiogenesis in matrigel, collagen, fibrin, and plasma clot. In Vitro Cell Dev Biol 1990;26(2):119–28.

[24] Zhu WH, Nicosia RF. The thin prep rat aortic ring assay: a modified method for the characterization of angiogenesis in whole mounts. Angiogenesis 2002;5(1–2):81–6.

[25] Mousa SA, O'Connor L, Davis FB, Davis PJ. Proangiogenesis action of the thyroid hormone analog 3,5-diiodothyropropionic acid (DITPA) is initiated at the cell surface and is integrin mediated. Endocrinology 2006;147(4):1602–7.

[26] Arnaoutova I, George J, Kleinman HK, Benton G. The endothelial cell tube formation assay on basement membrane turns 20: state of the science and the art. Angiogenesis 2009;12(3):267–74.

[27] Kubota Y, Kleinman HK, Martin GR, Lawley TJ. Role of laminin and basement membrane in the morphological differentiation of human endothelial cells into capillary-like structures. J Cell Biol 1988;107(4):1589–98.

[28] Donovan D, Brown NJ, Bishop ET, Lewis CE. Comparison of three in vitro human 'angiogenesis' assays with capillaries formed in vivo. Angiogenesis 2001;4(2):113–21.

[29] Zhou J, Wang H, Zhang H, Lutz AM, Tian L, Hristov D, Willmann JK. VEGFR2-targeted three-dimensional ultrasound imaging can predict responses to anti-angiogenic therapy in preclinical models of colon cancer. Cancer Res 2016;76(14):4081–9.

[30] Phillips PG, Birnby LM. Nitric oxide modulates caveolin-1 and matrix metalloproteinase-9 expression and distribution at the endothelial cell/tumor cell interface. Am J Physiol Lung Cell Mol Physiol 2004;286(5):L1055–65.

[31] Phillips PG, Birnby LM, Narendran A, Milonovich WL. Nitric oxide modulates capillary formation at the endothelial cell-tumor cell interface. Am J Physiol Lung Cell Mol Physiol 2001;281(1):L278–90.

[32] Lincoln DW 2nd, Phillips PG. Bove K. Estrogen-induced Ets-1 promotes capillary formation in an in vitro tumor angiogenesis model. Breast Cancer Res Treat 2003;78(2):167–78.

[33] Hetheridge C, Mavria G, Mellor H. Uses of the in vitro endothelial-fibroblast organotypic co-culture assay in angiogenesis research. Biochem Soc Trans 2011;39(6):1597–600.

[34] Nguyen D, Akay YM, Akay M. Investigating glioblastoma angiogenesis using a 3D in vitro GeIma microwell platform. IEEE Trans Nanobioscience 2016;15(3):289–93.

[35] Colman RW, Jameson BA, Lin Y, Johnson D, Mousa SA. Domain 5 of high molecular weight kininogen (kininostatin) down-regulates endothelial cell proliferation and migration and inhibits angiogenesis. Blood 2000;95(2):543–50.

[36] Wessels JT, Busse AC, Mahrt J, Dullin C, Grabbe E, Mueller GA. In vivo imaging in experimental preclinical tumor research—a review. Cytometry A 2007;71(8):542–9.

CHAPTER 3

Anti-Angiogenesis in Multiple Myeloma

Domenico Ribatti and Angelo Vacca

Contents

ANGIOGENESIS IN MULTIPLE MYELOMA

Multiple myeloma (MM) is characterized by uncontrolled proliferation of malignant plasma cells that infiltrate the bone marrow and is usually preceded by a premalignant stage named monoclonal gammopathy of undetermined significance (MGUS), which progresses to overt MM. The history of treatment of MM begins in the 1960s, when melphalan plus prednisone was introduced and achieved median survival of 2–3 years. MM is still incurable despite the implementation of novel therapies and the majority of patients relapse even if initially they respond to therapy.

In MM microvascular density increases with progression and is related with the plasma cell labeling index. Angiogenesis favors expansion of the MM mass by promoting plasma cell proliferation [1]. Myeloma plasma cells induce angiogenesis through the secretion of vascular endothelial growth factor (VEGF), fibroblast growth factor-2 (FGF2), matrix metalloproteinase-2 and -9 (MMP-2 and MMP-9), and by induction of host inflammatory cell infiltration [1].

Anti-Angiogenesis Strategies in Cancer Therapies
http://dx.doi.org/10.1016/B978-0-12-802576-5.00003-6

Interactions between plasma cells, hematopoietic stem cells, fibroblasts, osteoblasts/osteoclasts, chondroclasts, endothelial cells, endothelial cell progenitor cells, T cells, macrophages, and mast cells occur [2].

We have demonstrated that macrophages, mast cells, and fibroblasts contribute to angiogenesis in active MM, and this ability proceeds parallel to progression of the plasma cell tumors [3–5].

The VEGF signaling pathway can be inhibited in MM at various levels, that is, by blocking the activity of VEGF with monoclonal antibodies, blocking the VEGF receptors (VEGFRs) with specific inhibitors, or interfering with the tyrosine kinases activated by the VEGF/VEGFR interactions [6].

THALIDOMIDE AND ITS ANALOGS

Thalidomide was first used as a sedative and hypnotic drug in 1950s and was withdrawn from the market due to its teratogenic effects [7]. Thalidomide and its analogs lenalidomide and pomalidomide are designed as immunomodulatory drugs (IMiDs). Pomalidomide is the most potent IMiD, having 100 times the strength of thalidomide and 10 times that of lenalidomide [8].

We have studied the anti-angiogenic properties of thalidomide in MM endothelial cells and demonstrated that therapeutic doses of thalidomide markedly downregulate key angiogenic genes in a dose-dependent manner. Moreover, secretion of VEGF, FGF2, and hepatocyte growth factor (HGF) also diminished dose-dependently in culture-conditioned media of active MM endothelial cells [9]. Moreover, thalidomide enhances T-cell- and natural killer (NK)-cell-mediated immunological responses, induces caspase-8 mediated apoptosis and downregulates interleukin-6 (IL-6) production within the bone marrow microenvironment [10,11]. The immune-modulatory effect of thalidomide and IMiDs is recognized as a major determinant of their anti-MM activity [10].

Singhal and coworkers for the first time used thalidomide on compassionate basis to treat 84 patients with relapsed and refractory MM and found it remarkably effective with a response rate of 32% [12]. Several clinical studies were led in 2006 by the Food and Drug Administration (FDA) for the approval of the drug in patients with relapsed/refractory MM and this led to response rates as high as 65% [13–15].

Lenalidomide is an analog of thalidomide with anti-angiogenic proprieties. It inhibits VEGF-induced PI3-K-Akt pathway signaling and hypoxia inducible factor 1 alpha (HIF-1α) expression [16], exerts anti-tumor necrosis factor alpha (TNF-α) activity, modulates the immune response stimulating T-cells' and NK-cells' activities, induces apoptosis of tumor cells and decreases the binding of MM cells to bone marrow stromal components [10,11,17,18].

We have demonstrated that a clinically achievable concentration of lenalidomide is anti-angiogenic in vivo and inhibits MM endothelial cells' migration (Fig. 3.1) [19]. Lenalidomide downregulates key angiogenic genes and VEGF/VEGFR-2-mediated downstream signaling pathways involved in cell motility and nuclear factor kappa B (NFκB). Moreover, a proteomic analysis reveals that lenalidomide-treated MM endothelial cells modulate the expression levels of angiogenesis-related genes controlling MM endothelial cell motility and invasiveness, cell shape and cytoskeletal dynamic remodeling, as well as energy metabolism pathways and protein clearance [19].

In 2006, lenalidomide received FDA approval for the treatment of MM patients who have received at least one prior therapy. A phase III clinical trial using lenalidomide in combination with dexamethasone in newly diagnosed patients has been completed and showed that lenalidomide plus low-dose dexamethasone is associated with superior overall survival compared to lenalidomide plus high-dose dexamethasone [20].

BORTEZOMIB

Bortezomib is a proteasome inhibitor that induces endothelial cell apoptosis [21], inhibits VEGF, IL-6, angiopoietin-1 and -2 (Ang-1 and Ang-2) and insulin-like growth factor-1 (IGF-1) secretion in bone marrow stromal cells and MM endothelial cells [22,23] and HIF-1α activity [24]. Roccaro and coworkers have demonstrated

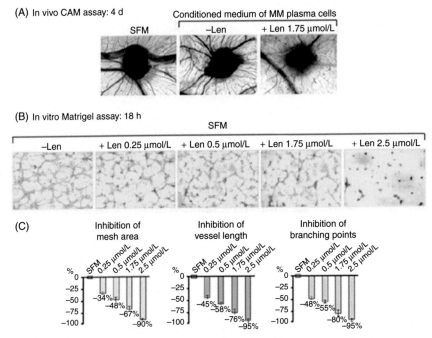

Figure 3.1 *Lenalidomide inhibits angiogenesis in chorioallantoic membrane (CAM) and Matrigel.* (A) CAMs were incubated with gelatin sponges loaded with SFM (left) and with conditioned medium of multiple myeloma (MM) plasma cells either alone (middle) or supplemented with 1.75 mmol/L lenalidomide (right). Note the inhibition of MM angiogenesis by the drug. (B) lenalidomide inhibits multiple myeloma endothelial cells (MMEC) angiogenesis in the Matrigel in a dose-dependent manner. MMECs arranged to form a closely knit capillary-like plexus (left), whereas the tube formation was gradually blocked with increasing lenalidomide doses with a full inhibition at 2.5 mmol/L (right). A representative patient is shown. (C) skeletonization of the mesh was followed by measurements of its topological parameters: mesh area, vessel length, and branching points. Data are presented as mean ±SD of percent inhibition. *Len,* lenalidomide; *SFM,* serum free medium. *(Reproduced from De Luisi A, Ferrucci A, Coluccia AM, Ria R, Moschetta M, de Luca E, Pieroni L, Maffia M, Urbani A, Di Pietro G, Guarini A, Ranieri G, Ditonno P, Berardi S, Caivano A, Basile A, Cascavilla N, Capalbo S, Quarta G, Dammacco F, Ribatti D, Vacca A. Lenalidomide restrains motility and overangiogenic potential of bone marrow endothelial cells in patients with active multiple myeloma. Clin Cancer Res 2011;17(7):1935–1946).*

RPMI (neg. control)   FGF-2 (pos. control)   Bortezomib

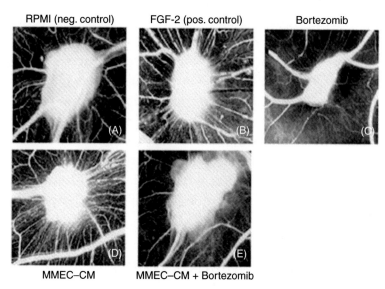

MMEC–CM   MMEC–CM + Bortezomib

Figure 3.2 *Bortezomib inhibits angiogenesis in vivo in the CAM assay.* The CAM was incubated with a gelatin sponge loaded with RPMI (A), 200 Ag/mL FGF-2 (B), 20 nmol/L bortezomib (C), and with multiple myeloma endothelial cell (MMEC) conditioned media (CM) either alone (D) or with 20 nmol/L bortezomib (E). Bortezomib significantly inhibited basal angiogenesis induced by sponges loaded with vehicle alone (C). Moreover, CAM implanted with FGF-2 (B) or with MMEC conditioned media (D) increased macroscopic vessel counts. Bortezomib significantly inhibited MMEC CM–induced angiogenesis (E), evidenced both by macroscopic vessel counts and by the number of eggs out of total with >50% inhibition in the angiogenic response compared with vehicle. *FGF-2*, Fibroblast growth factor-2; *RPMI*, Roswell Park Memorial Institute. *(Reproduced from Roccaro AM, Hideshima T, Raje N, Kumar S, Ishitsuka K, Yasui H, Shiraishi N, Ribatti D, Nico B, Vacca A, Dammacco F, Richardson PG, Anderson KC. Bortezomib mediates antiangiogenesis in multiple myeloma via direct and indirect effects on endothelial cells. Cancer Res 2006;66(1):184–191).*

that bortezomib inhibits the proliferation of MM endothelial cells in a dose- and time-dependent manner [22]. Moreover, in functional assays of angiogenesis, including chemotaxis, adhesion to fibronectin, capillary formation on Matrigel, and chorioallantoic membrane (CAM) assay (Fig. 3.2), bortezomib inhibited angiogenesis in a dose-dependent manner.

Bortezomib was approved by the FDA in 2005. The combination of bortezomib, thalidomide, and dexamethasone in patients with relapsed MM showed an overall response rate of 70% including near complete response in 16% of patients [25]. In addition, the combination of bortezomib, melphalan, and prednisone in nontransplant candidates resulted in an overall response rate of 89% [26].

Second-generation proteasome inhibitors can overcome bortezomib resistance in preclinical models. Carfilzomib results in increased extent and duration of inhibition compared with bortezomib [27].

TYROSINE KINASE INHIBITORS (TKIs)

Vatalanib, an orally administered broad-spectrum TKI, inhibited proliferation and migration of MM cells [28], while imatinib mesylate blocked cell-cycle progression in MM and potentiated the effects of conventional anti-myeloma agents in vitro [29]. Sorafenib exerted a significant anti-myeloma activity and synergized with common anti-myeloma drugs [30]. A constitutive activation of two dasatinib targets, platelet derived growth factor receptor beta (PDGFRβ)/Src, has been demonstrated in plasma cells and endothelial cells isolated from patients with MM [31]. Moreover, dasatinib significantly delayed MM tumor growth and angiogenesis in vivo, showing a synergistic cytotoxicity with melphalan, prednisone, bortezomib, and thalidomide [32].

ZOLEDRONIC ACID

We have demonstrated that therapeutic doses of zoledronic acid markedly inhibit in vitro proliferation, chemotaxis, and capillarogenesis of MM endothelial cells and in vivo angiogenesis in the CAM assay [33]. These effects are partly sustained by gene and protein inhibition of VEGF and VEGFR-2 in an autocrine loop. These data suggest that the zoledronic acid anti-tumoral activity in MM is also sustained by anti-angiogenesis, which would partly account for its therapeutic efficacy in MM [34]. Moreover, we have demonstrated that bortezomib and zoledronic acid display distinct and synergistic inhibitory effects on cell proliferation, adhesion, migration, and expression of angiogenic cytokines by MM macrophages [35]. These data provide evidence that the exposure of bone marrow macrophages in MM during the treatment with zoledronic acid and bortezomib, alone and/or in combination, impacts their angiogenic properties.

CONCLUSIONS

The median survival for patients with MM has almost doubled since the introduction of thalidomide, lenalidomide and bortezomib [36]. Both thalidomide and bortezomib showed response rates of 30–40% when used as monotherapy in relapsed patients. However, when combined with steroids or alkylating agents, the response rates double. These agents have been incorporated into conventional cytotoxic and transplantation regimens and used as a treatment for newly diagnosed MM. Together with IMiDs and dexamethasone, bortezomib is now integrated as frontline therapy in the majority of patients, with overall response rates as high 100% with lenalidomide/bortezomib/dexamethasone [37]. Nevertheless, most patients still relapse after an initial response to treatment and multidrug resistance often emerges over time [36].

The principal drawback in the management of anti-angiogenic drugs in the treatment of MM is that several angiogenic molecules may be synthesized by tumor cells, and that tumor cells may depend on different factors for its supply.

A very common side effect of anti-angiogenic therapy is hypertension, which is associated with nitric oxide changes, pruning of normal vessels, as well as effects on renal salt homeostasis. Toxic peripheral neuropathy represents a dose-limiting debilitating side effect of the treatment of MM with thalidomide, bortezomib and lenalidomide.

Further studies to optimize treatment regimens and to increase our understanding of tumor angiogenesis and the mechanisms underlying the development of resistance are required.

ACKNOWLEDGMENTS

The research leading to these results received funding from the European Union Seventh Framework Programme (FP7/2007-2013) under grant agreement 278570 to DR and 278706 to AV.

REFERENCES

[1] Vacca A, Ribatti D. Bone marrow angiogenesis in multiple myeloma. Leukemia 2006;20(2):193–9.
[2] Ribatti D, Nico B, Vacca A. Importance of the bone marrow microenvironment in inducing the angiogenic response in multiple myeloma. Oncogene 2006;25(31):4257–66.
[3] Scavelli C, Nico B, Cirulli T, Ria R, Di Pietro G, Mangieri D, Bacigalupo A, Mangialardi G, Coluccia AML, Caravita T, Molica S, Ribatti D, Dammacco F, Vacca A. Vasculogenic mimicry by bone marrow macrophages in patients with multiple myeloma. Oncogene 2008;27(5):663–74.
[4] Nico B, Mangieri D, Crivellato E, Vacca A, Ribatti D. Mast cells contribute to vasculogenic mimicry in multiple myeloma. Stem Cells Dev 2008;17(1):19–22.
[5] Frassanito MA, Rao L, Moschetta M, Ria R, Di Marzo L, De Luisi A, Racanelli V, Catacchio I, Berardi S, Basile A, Menu E, Ruggieri S, Nico B, Ribatti D, Fumarulo R, Dammacco F, Vanderkerken K, Vacca A. Bone marrow fibroblasts parallel multiple myeloma progression in patients and mice: in vitro and in vivo studies. Leukemia 2014;28(4):904–16.
[6] Ria R, Roccaro AM, Merchionne F, Vacca A, Dammacco F, Ribatti D. Vascular endothelial growth factor and its receptors in multiple myeloma. Leukemia 2003;17(10):1961–6.
[7] Ribatti D, Vacca A. Therapeutic renaissance of thalidomide in the treatment of haematological malignancies. Leukemia 2005;19(9):1525–31.
[8] Gertz MA. Pomalidomide and myeloma meningitis. Leuk Lymphoma 2013;54(4):681–2.
[9] Vacca A, Scavelli C, Montefusco V, Di Pietro G, Neri A, Mattioli M, Bicciato S, Nico B, Ribatti D, Dammacco F, Corradini P. Thalidomide downregulates angiogenic genes in bone marrow endothelial cells of patients with active multiple myeloma. J Clin Oncol 2005;23(23):5334–46.

[10] Davies FE, Raje N, Hideshima T, Lentzsch S, Young G, Tai YT, Lin B, Podar K, Gupta D, Chauhan D, Treon SP, Richardson PG, Schlossman RL, Morgan GJ, Muller GW, Stirling DI, Anderson KC. Thalidomide and immunomodulatory derivatives augment natural killer cell cytotoxicity in multiple myeloma. Blood 2001;98(1):210–6.

[11] Mitsiades N, Mitsiades CS, Poulaki V, Chauhan D, Richardson PG, Hideshima T, Munshi NC, Treon SP, Anderson KC. Apoptotic signaling induced by immunomodulatory thalidomide analogs in human multiple myeloma cells: therapeutic implications. Blood 2002;99(12):4525–30.

[12] Singhal S, Mehta J, Desikan R, Ayers D, Roberson P, Eddlemon P, Munshi N, Anaissie E, Wilson C, Dhodapkar M, Zeddis J, Barlogie B. Antitumor activity of thalidomide in refractory multiple myeloma. N Engl J Med 1999;341(21):1565–71.

[13] Rajkumar SV, Blood E, Vesole D, Fonseca R, Greipp PR. Phase III clinical trial of thalidomide plus dexamethasone compared with dexamethasone alone in newly diagnosed multiple myeloma: a clinical trial coordinated by the Eastern Cooperative Oncology Group. J Clin Oncol 2006;24(3):431–6.

[14] Rajkumar SV, Fonseca R, Dispenzieri A, Lacy MQ, Lust JA, Witzig TE, Kyle RA, Gertz MA, Greipp PR. Thalidomide in the treatment of relapsed multiple myeloma. Mayo Clin Proc 2000;75(9):897–901.

[15] Rajkumar SV, Rosinol L, Hussein M, Catalano J, Jedrzejczak W, Lucy L, Olesnyckyj M, Yu Z, Knight R, Zeldis JB, Blade J. Multicenter, randomized, double-blind, placebo-controlled study of thalidomide plus dexamethasone compared with dexamethasone as initial therapy for newly diagnosed multiple myeloma. J Clin Oncol 2008;26(13):2171–7.

[16] Lu L, Payvandi F, Wu L, Zhang LH, Hariri RJ, Man HW, Chen RS, Muller GW, Hughes CC, Stirling DI, Schafer PH, Bartlett JB. The anti-cancer drug lenalidomide inhibits angiogenesis and metastasis via multiple inhibitory effects on endothelial cell function in normoxic and hypoxic conditions. Microvasc Res 2009;77(2):78–86.

[17] Dredge K, Horsfall R, Robinson SP, Zhang LH, Lu L, Tang Y, Shirley MA, Muller G, Schafer P, Stirling D, Dalgleish AG, Bartlett JB. Orally administered lenalidomide (CC-5013) is anti-angiogenic in vivo and inhibits endothelial cell migration and Akt phosphorylation in vitro. Microvasc Res 2005;69(1–2):56–63.

[18] Chang DH, Liu N, Klimek V, Hassoun H, Mazumder A, Nimer SD, Jagannath S, Dhodapkar MV. Enhancement of ligand-dependent activation of human natural killer T cells by lenalidomide: therapeutic implications. Blood 2006;108(2):618–21.

[19] De Luisi A, Ferrucci A, Coluccia AM, Ria R, Moschetta M, de Luca E, Pieroni L, Maffia M, Urbani A, Di Pietro G, Guarini A, Ranieri G, Ditonno P, Berardi S, Caivano A, Basile A, Cascavilla N, Capalbo S, Quarta G, Dammacco F, Ribatti D, Vacca A. Lenalidomide restrains motility and overangiogenic potential of bone marrow endothelial cells in patients with active multiple myeloma. Clin Cancer Res 2011;17(7):1935–46.

[20] Chen C, Reece DE, Siegel D, Niesvizky R, Boccia RV, Stadtmauer EA, Abonour R, Richardson P, Matous J, Kumar S, Bahlis NJ, Alsina M, Vescio R, Coutre SE, Pietronigro D, Knight RD, Zeldis JB, Rajkumar V. Expanded safety experience with lenalidomide plus dexamethasone in relapsed or refractory multiple myeloma. Br J Haematol 2009;146(2):164–70.

[21] Williams S, Pettaway C, Song R, Papandreou C, Logothetis C, McConkey DJ. Differential effects of the proteasome inhibitor bortezomib on apoptosis and angiogenesis in human prostate tumor xenografts. Mol Cancer Ther 2003;2(9):835–43.

[22] Roccaro AM, Hideshima T, Raje N, Kumar S, Ishitsuka K, Yasui H, Shiraishi N, Ribatti D, Nico B, Vacca A, Dammacco F, Richardson PG, Anderson KC. Bortezomib mediates antiangiogenesis in multiple myeloma via direct and indirect effects on endothelial cells. Cancer Res 2006;66(1):184–91.

[23] Hideshima T, Chauhan D, Hayashi T, Akiyama M, Mitsiades N, Mitsiades C, Podar K, Munshi NC, Richardson PG, Anderson KC. Proteasome inhibitor PS-341 abrogates IL-6 triggered signaling cascades via caspase-dependent downregulation of gp130 in multiple myeloma. Oncogene 2003;22(52):8386–93.

[24] Shin DH, Chun YS, Lee DS, Huang LE, Park JW. Bortezomib inhibits tumor adaptation to hypoxia by stimulating the FIH-mediated repression of hypoxia-inducible factor-1. Blood 2008;111(6):3131–6.

[25] Richardson PG, Mitsiades C, Ghobrial I, Anderson K. Beyond single-agent bortezomib: combination regimens in relapsed multiple myeloma. Curr Opin Oncol 2006;18(6):598–608.

[26] Mateos MV, Hernandez JM, Hernandez MT, Gutierrez NC, Palomera L, Fuertes M, Diaz-Mediavilla J, Lahuerta JJ, de la Rubia J, Terol MJ, Sureda A, Bargay J, Ribas P, de Arriba F, Alegre A, Oriol A, Carrera D, Garcia-Larana J, Garcia-Sanz R, Blade J, Prosper F, Mateo G, Esseltine DL, van de Velde H, San Miguel JF. Bortezomib plus melphalan and prednisone in elderly untreated patients with multiple myeloma: results of a multicenter phase 1/2 study. Blood 2006;108(7):2165–72.

[27] Kuhn DJ, Orlowski RZ, Bjorklund CC. Second generation proteasome inhibitors: carfilzomib and immunoproteasome-specific inhibitors (IPSIs). Curr Cancer Drug Targets 2011;11(3):285–95.

[28] Lin B, Podar K, Gupta D, Tai YT, Li S, Weller E, Hideshima T, Lentzsch S, Davies F, Li C, Weisberg E, Schlossman RL, Richardson PG, Griffin JD, Wood J, Munshi NC, Anderson KC. The vascular endothelial growth factor receptor tyrosine kinase inhibitor PTK787/ZK222584 inhibits growth and migration of multiple myeloma cells in the bone marrow microenvironment. Cancer Res 2002;62(17):5019–26.

[29] Pandiella A, Carvajal-Vergara X, Tabera S, Mateo G, Gutierrez N, San Miguel JF. Imatinib mesylate (STI571) inhibits multiple myeloma cell pro-liferation and potentiates the effect of common antimyeloma agents. Br J Haematol 2003;123(5):858–68.

[30] Ramakrishnan V, Timm M, Haug JL, Kimlinger TK, Wellik LE, Witzig TE, Rajkumar SV, Adjei AA, Kumar S. Sorafenib, a dual Raf kinase/vascular endothelial growth factor receptor inhibitor has significant anti-myeloma activity and synergizes with common anti-myeloma drugs. Oncogene 2010;29(8):1190–202.

[31] Coluccia AM, Cirulli T, Neri P, Mangieri D, Colanardi MC, Gnoni A, Di Renzo N, Dammacco F, Tassone P, Ribatti D, Gambacorti-Passerini C, Vacca A. Validation of PDGFRβ and c-Src tyrosine kinases as tumor/vessel targets in patients with multiple myeloma: preclinical efficacy of the novel, orally available inhibitor dasatinib. Blood 2008;112(4):1346–56.

[32] de Queiroz Crusoe E, Maiso P, Fernandez-Lazaro D, San-Segundo L, Ga-rayoa M, Garcia-Gomez A, Gutierrez NC, Delgado M, Colado E, Martin-Sanchez J, Lee FY, Ocio EM. Transcriptomic rationale for the synergy observed with dasatinib+bortezomib+dexamethasone in multiple my-eloma. Ann Hematol 2012;91(2):257–69.

[33] Scavelli C, Di Pietro G, Cirulli T, Coluccia M, Boccarelli A, Giannini T, Mangialardi G, Bertieri R, Coluccia AML, Ribatti D, Dammacco F, Vacca A. Zoledronic acid affects over-angiogenic phenotype of endothelial cells in patients with multiple myeloma. Mol Cancer Ther 2007;6(12):3256–62.

[34] Henk HJ, Teitelbaum A, Perez JR, Kaura S. Persistency with zoledronic acid is associated with clinical benefit in patients with multiple myeloma. Am J Hematol 2012;87(5):490–5.

[35] Moschetta M, Di Pietro G, Ria R, Gnoni A, Mangialardi G, Guarini A, Ditonno P, Musto P, D'Auria F, Ricciardi MR, Dammacco F, Ribatti D, Vacca A. Bortezomib and zoledronic acid on angiogenic and vasculogenic activities of bone marrow macrophages in patients with multiple myelo-ma. Eur J Cancer 2010;46(2):420–9.

[36] Anderson KC. The 39th David A. Karnofsky Lecture: bench-to-bedside translation of targeted therapies in multiple myeloma. J Clin Oncol 2012;30(4):445–52.

[37] Richardson PG, Weller E, Lonial S, Jakubowiak AJ, Jagannath S, Raje NS, Avigan DE, Xie W, Ghobrial IM, Schlossman RL, Mazumder A, Munshi NC, Vesole DH, Joyce R, Kaufman JL, Doss D, Warren DL, Lunde LE, Kaster S, Delaney C, Hideshima T, Mitsiades CS, Knight R, Esseltine DL, Anderson KC. Lenalidomide, bortezomib, and dexamethasone combination therapy in patients with newly diagnosed multiple myeloma. Blood 2010;116(5):679–86.

CHAPTER 4

Interface between Thrombosis, Inflammation, and Angiogenesis in Cancer Progression

Shaker A. Mousa, Vandhana Muralidharan-Chari and Paul J. Davis

Contents

CANCER-ASSOCIATED THROMBOSIS

Cancer cells exploit fundamental physiological mechanisms for their survival and progression. Specifically during cancer progression, tumor cells successfully engage and orchestrate the hemostatic system, with a resulting clinical diagnosis of Trousseau's syndrome. In 1865, Armand Trousseau made a shrewd clinical observation of blood hypercoagulation in cancer patients, namely, that the presence of an unexpected migratory thrombophlebitis heralds occult visceral malignancy. This thrombotic condition is frequently associated with chronic intravascular coagulopathy, platelet-rich microthrombi, microangiopathic hemolytic anemia, verrucous endocarditis, and deep vein thrombosis [1,2]. Tumor type-specific oncogenic transformations cause upregulation of a protein called tissue factor (TF) on tumor cells.

During the early phase of cancer progression, TF that is present on tumor cells enables local thrombin generation, initiating fibrin

Anti-Angiogenesis Strategies in Cancer Therapies
http://dx.doi.org/10.1016/B978-0-12-802576-5.00004-8

51

deposition and recruitment of platelets through protease–activated receptor (PAR) signaling. This localized process enables tumor cells to have increased attachment and firm adhesion, in addition to protecting them from elimination by natural killer cells. TF-PAR signaling has also been shown to initiate signaling to promote angiogenesis [3]. All of these events are pivotal to cancer progression, culminating in an advanced stage of cancer characterized by the hypercoagulable state [4]. TF is also expressed by epithelial cells, macrophages and other cell types that are normally separated from blood and circulating coagulation factors. However, low levels of TF are seen on circulating monocytes and leukocyte-derived microparticles and on cytokine-stimulated endothelial cells, which can be concentrated at sites of injury or local inflammation [5–7].

The coagulation, fibrinolysis, and platelet systems that are involved in thrombosis and hemostasis play a key role in angiogenesis modulation. A close association between inflammation and thrombosis in the regulation of angiogenesis is well established [8–10]. As such for successful tumor progression, the dynamic interplay of thrombosis, angiogenesis, and inflammation is the result of downstream signaling events emanating from a key coordinator molecule, TF, complexed with Factor VIIa, Factor Xa, and PAR (VIIa–Xa–PAR, Fig. 4.1).

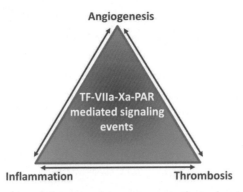

Figure 4.1 *Interplay of the vascular processes, thrombosis, inflammation and angiogenesis regulated by signaling events triggered by TF-VIIa-Xa-PAR.* Abbreviations: *VIIa*, Factor VIIa; *PAR*, protease-activated receptor; *TF*, tissue factor; *Xa*, Factor Xa.

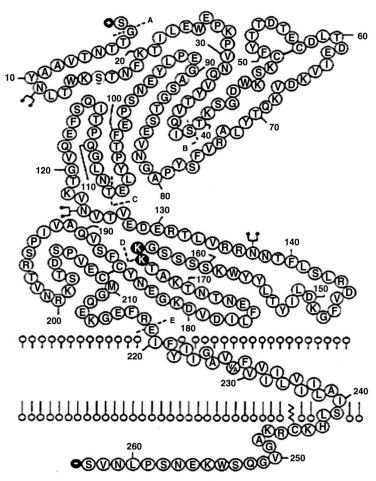

Figure 4.2 *Structure of tissue factor (TF).* The single-letter amino acid code is used to identify amino acids. Sites of carbohydrate attachment are represented by two *darkened circles* connected by a single bar to the amino acid. *(Reprinted with permission from Mody RS, Carson SD. Tissue factor cytoplasmic domain peptide is multiply phosphorylated in vitro. Biochemistry 1997;36(25):7869-7875 [11]. Copyright 1997 American Chemical Society).*

TF (also called CD412) is a Type II cytokine receptor, is 2630 amino acids long and weighs 46 kDa. This membrane-integral glycoprotein has 219 amino acids at the N-terminus that are extracellular, 23 amino acids that form the transmembrane domain and 21 amino acids at the C-terminus that are intracellular [11] (Fig. 4.2).

TF initiates the extrinsic coagulation cascade and enables blood co-agulation, thrombin (Factor IIa) generation, and thrombus formation [12]. In the event of vascular injury, TF serves to provide hemostatic balance around blood vessels by activating the proteases in the coagu-lation cascade to produce an effective fibrin clot. It also functions as a receptor and a cofactor for activated Factor VII (FVIIa) to initiate blood coagulation by formation of the TF-VIIa complex [13]. Proco-agulant activity is localized in the extracellular domain of TF [14]. The cytoplasmic domain, which is not required for procoagulant function, contains three serine residues that can be phosphorylated [11,15]. The coagulation cascade proceeds with the sequential generation of coagulant mediators (FVIIa, FXa, and FIIa: active serine proteases) and fibrin production, all of which are proinflammatory [16].

In addition to its seemingly simple role in the coagulation cascade, TF facilitates signaling events in vascular cells that con-tribute to various biological processes, including angiogenesis and inflammation (Fig. 4.3). The signaling is mediated by the activation of PARs by the coagulation proteases FVIIa, FXa, and thrombin [17–19]. Four PARs (PARs 1 through 4) have been described [20]. PARs 1, 3, and 4 are activated by thrombin. PAR2, however, is unique in that it is activated by trypsin [21] and by the TF-VIIa complex and FXa [22], rather than by thrombin. In addition to their presence on normal cells, PAR1 and PAR2 have been identi-fied on a wide variety of tumor cells [23–29].

In addition to the activity of thrombin during the initial ar-rest of metastasizing tumor cells, other coagulation proteases gen-erated during tumor progression function as alternative activators of PAR1, including FXa [30,31], plasmin [32,33], activated protein C [34,35], tissue kallikreins [36,37], and matrix metalloproteinases 1 [38]. PAR2, originally cloned as a receptor cleavable by trypsin and not by thrombin, is activated by coagulation protease factors VIIa and Xa [22,39], tissue kallikreins [40], and membrane-type serine proteases [41–43]. A growing body of evidence indicates that signaling by PARs—initiated specifically by tumor cell-expressed TF-VIIa—plays a critical role in angiogenesis and inflammation.

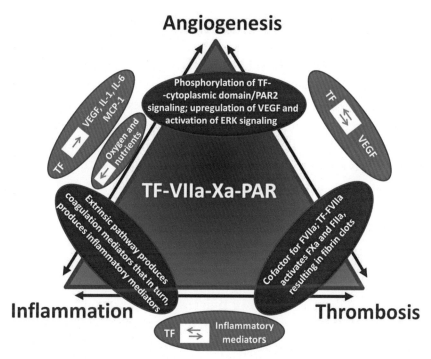

Figure 4.3 *Illustration of the role of TF-VIIa-Xa-PAR in thrombosis, angiogenesis, and inflammation.* Feedback between angiogenesis and inflammation; inflammation and thrombosis and thrombosis and angiogenesis are facilitated by TF-VIIa-Xa-PAR signaling downstream events. Abbreviations: *IIa*, Factor IIa; *VIIa*, Factor VIIa; *IL*, interleukin; *MCP-1*, monocyte chemoattractant protein; *PAR*, protease-activated receptor; *TF*, tissue factor; *VEGF*, vascular endothelial growth factor; *Xa*, Factor Xa.

The TF-VIIa complex activates both PAR2 and coagulation protease FXa, while still assembled in the transient ternary TF-VIIa–Xa complex and initiates signaling events through PAR1 or PAR2. TF-VIIa–induced tumor-associated hypercoagulation and resulting thrombotic events require the generation of thrombin. In contrast, TF-VIIa–induced angiogenesis and inflammation do not necessarily require thrombin generation. This would rather require upregulation of growth factors, such as vascular endothelial growth factor (VEGF) and other processes. Here, we will focus on the signaling events mediated by TF-VIIa–Xa ternary complex via PAR2 to promote angiogenesis and inflammation during cancer progression.

TF-VIIa-PAR2 SIGNALING REGULATES ANGIOGENESIS

In animal models, inhibitors of TF–VIIa suppress tumor growth and in vivo angiogenesis, whereas potent anti-coagulants that inhibit FXa display no such activity [44]. Studies also show that use of anti-coagulants, such as heparin regulates angiogenesis and tumor growth [45–47]. Since the hemostatic activity mediated by TF–FVIIa is mediated through the activation of FXa, this indicates that proteolytic activity of TF–FVIIa promotes tumor growth and angiogenesis through a novel proangiogenic mechanism and independently of hemostasis.

Indeed, activation of PAR2 by TF–VIIa results in G-protein coupled receptor signaling events mediated via G-proteins, such as $G\alpha12/13$, $G\alpha q$, and $G\alpha i$ as well as G-protein independent signaling through recruitment of β-arrestin leading to promigratory ERK and cofilin activation [48,49]. A comprehensive gene profiling study compared the genes induced by TF–VIIa-PAR2 signaling in breast cancer cells [50] with the direct activation of the thrombin receptor PAR1. This investigation identified genes induced by TF–VIIa signaling, including *PAI-1*, *Cyr61*, *uPA*. In addition, TF–VIIa also induced proangiogenic chemokines and growth factors, such as interleukin-8 (IL-8), CXCL1, VEGF, and immune regulators including granulocyte-macrophage colony stimulating factor and macrophage colony stimulating factor. Both of the latter factors are crucial for the recruitment and differentiation of myeloid cell populations in the tumor microenvironment. Thus, TF–VIIa-PAR2 signaling in cancer cells promotes angiogenesis and influences innate immune cells vital for tumor progression and metastasis.

In knock-in mice that lack the TF cytoplasmic domain, it was found that transplanted syngeneic tumors grew ~twofold faster in these mice, compared to wild type controls. This suggests that TF cytoplasmic domain in host cells plays a negative regulatory role in tumor angiogenesis [3]. Furthermore, deletion of PAR2 in these mice did not affect angiogenesis, that is, angiogenesis was comparable to that in wild type mice. These results raise the issue of how the cytoplasmic domain of TF-mediated inhibition of angiogenesis is regulated in physiological and pathological conditions. The answer came from two studies [51,52]. By default, the cytoplasmic domain of TF remains unphosphorylated in endothelial cells and activation of protein kinase C alpha (PKC-α) triggers phosphorylation, which is activated by PAR1 signaling and not by PAR2 signaling (Fig. 4.3). Activation of phosphatidylcholine-specific phospholipase C occurs upstream of PKC-α and accounts for this unique signaling response by PAR2. Thioester modification of the cytoplasmic cysteine counteracts TF phosphorylation. Thus PAR2 expression and changes in palmitoylation status of TF are the key regulators of TF cytoplasmic domain phosphorylation. Detection of PAR2 in pathological blood vessels suggests that TF phosphorylation in the context of PAR2 signaling may switch off the suppressive function of the TF cytoplasmic domain that enables PAR2 dependent pathological angiogenesis.

Extracellular signal-related kinases (ERK1/2) are activated by the TF-FVIIa interaction [53,54]. Activation of this pathway does not depend upon an intact cytoplasmic domain of TF in a kidney cell model [53]. In mouse fibroblasts, phosphoinositide 3-kinase (PI3-K) is activated upstream of ERK1/2 by TF-FVIIa [54]. It is also known that PI3-K activation may lead to p38-mitogen activated protein kinase (MAPK) activation via Rac, one of the small Rho-like GTPases [55]. The fact that PI3-K can be activated upstream of ERK1/2 does not mean that this is a requirement for the angiogenic response. The linkage of PI3-K to ERK1/2 may involve other cellular responses to TF-FVIIa activation or coordinated events, such as a combination of angiogenesis and inflammation. From Table 4.1, which summarizes studies of various signaling cascades activated by TF-VIIa, we may conclude that ERK1/2 activation, in contrast to the proinflammatory response, is frequently involved in the angiogenic response to VEGF gene expression. VEGF has been shown to increase the expression of TF (Fig. 4.3) [56,57].

Table 4.1 Signal transduction pathways that lead to VEGF gene expression

Cell	Stimulus	Signal transduction	References
Astrocytoma	Normoxia	ERK1/2	[58]
	Hypoxia	PI3-K	
VSMC	Interleukin-1	p38 kinase	[59]
Breast cancer	Heregulin β1	p38 kinase	[60]
Kidney	High glucose	ERK1/2; PKC	[61]
Glioblastoma	Acidic extracellular pH	ERK1/2;AP-1	[62]
Glioblastoma	Epidermal growth factor	Ras; PI3-K	[63]
Glioblastoma	Ionizing radiation	ERK1/2;AP-1	[64]
Retina	Stretch	PI3-K; PKC	[65]
Gastric vascular	Prostaglandin E_2	ERK1/2; JNK1	[66]
Fibroblasts	Normoxia	Ras; ERK1/2	[67]
	Hypoxia	ERK1/2	
Fibroblasts	Normoxia	ERK1/2	[68]
	Hypoxia	ERK1/2	
Colon cancer	Serum starvation	ERK1/2	[69]

Abbreviations: AP-1, Activator protein-1; JNK, c-Jun N-terminal kinase; PKC, protein kinase C; VSMC, vascular smooth muscle cell.

Recent studies in human endothelial cells have shown that TF induction by an immune modulator and proinflammatory cytokine interleukin-33 promoted angiogenesis [70–72], providing evidence to support a link between coagulation, inflammation, and angiogenesis.

TF-VIIa-PAR2 SIGNALING REGULATES INFLAMMATION

Connection between inflammation and cancer was identified by Rudolf Virchow in 1863, when he noticed the presence of leukocytes in neoplastic tissues [73]. Indeed in many cancers, the inflammatory process is a cofactor in carcinogenesis [74]. The cytokine network of several common tumors is rich in inflammatory cytokines, growth factors, and chemokines. Many of these cytokines and chemokines, such as tumor necrosis factor (TNF), IL-1 and IL-6 are inducible by hypoxia [75]. TF is also induced by hypoxia in tumor tissues [76].

Active serine-proteases (FIIa, FVIIa, and FXa) and fibrin clot produced by the TF-initiated extrinsic coagulation act through cell receptors to mediate diverse intracellular events, including the production of proinflammatory mediators including cytokines, adhesion molecules, growth factors, PARs, interleukins, NFκB, and Toll-like receptor [16]. Several lines of evidence indicate the presence of coagulation-dependent inflammation in vivo. PARs generally mediate inflammation derived from coagulant mediators and fibrin. TF hypercoagulability triggers autocrine and paracrine events to amplify events leading to a vicious cycle of thrombotic actions/coagulation-inflammation-thrombosis. Coagulation inducers trigger production of inflammatory mediators, and the latter in turn activate coagulation by inducing TF expression by blood mononuclear cells and, possibly, vascular endothelium. In turn, TF expression regulates the inflammatory response (Fig. 4.3).

The ability of TF-VIIa to trigger inflammation occurs either via PAR1 or PAR2. Although a deficiency of either PAR1 or PAR2 in one study had no effect on inflammation or survival of mice, a combination of thrombin inhibition in PAR2-deficient mice reduced both inflammation and mortality similar to low-TF mice [8]. This indicates that PAR1 and PAR2 may have overlapping roles that contributed to the link between TF-triggered coagulation and inflammation. TF-VIIa or TF-VIIa-Xa activates PAR1 and PAR2. PARs induce diverse inflammatory signals, including the cytokines, such as TNF-α [77], IL-1, IL-6 [78,79], adhesion molecules (E-selectin, ICAM-1, VCAM-1) [80], the chemokine MCP-1, and growth factors, such as VEGF [81]. The role of IL-1 [82–84], IL-6 [85–87], and MCP-1 [88–90] in promoting tumor has been confirmed by recent studies. Thus, the inflammatory mediators and VEGF produced by TF-VIIa or TF-VIIa-Xa promote tumor angiogenesis. In turn, angiogenesis supports inflammation by facilitating the supply of oxygen and nutrients for the metabolic needs of the cells present at the inflammatory sites (Fig. 4.3) [91].

TF-mediated inflammation does not require active coagulation. Small amounts of coagulation factors are sufficient to promote downstream signaling [22]. TF-VIIa has been shown to amplify the proinflammatory functions of macrophages, such as reactive oxygen species production, expression of major histocompatibility complex II (MHCII) and cell adhesion molecules both in vivo and in vitro [92].

ROLE OF TF-VIIa IN CELLULAR SIGNALING

In addition to the earlier understanding of TF-VIIa in thrombosis, angiogenesis, and inflammation, it has also been observed to induce an array of cellular events. TF-VIIa was shown to induce calcium fluxes in tumor cells and endothelial cells [93]. Subsequently, other investigators reported that TF-VIIa induces: tyrosine phosphorylation in monocytes [94]; activation of Src family members c-Src, Lyn, and Yes followed by stimulation of PI3-K and activation of c-Akt/protein kinase B, Rac, Cdc42, p44/p42 MAPK, and p38 MAPK in fibroblasts [54]; expression of poly-A polymerase in a fibroblast cell line [95]; increased expression of the urokinase receptor in a pancreatic tumor cell line [96]; activation of phospholipase C and chemotaxis in fibroblasts [97]; and upregulation of genes, such as *EGR-1*, *Cyr61*, and *Connective Tissue Growth Factor* [56,98]. However, the physiologic consequences of all of these signaling events, which require catalytically active factor VIIa, are not fully known.

CONCLUSIONS

The role of TF-VIIa-Xa-PAR in the interfaces of angiogenesis, thrombosis, and inflammation is fully documented and represents a potentially novel set of targets in cancer management when these three processes are activated.

REFERENCES

[1] Varki A. Trousseau's syndrome: multiple definitions and multiple mechanisms. Blood 2007;110(6):1723–9.

[2] Sack GH Jr, Levin J, Bell WR. Trousseau's syndrome and other manifestations of chronic disseminated coagulopathy in patients with neoplasms: clinical, pathophysiologic, and therapeutic features. Medicine (Baltimore) 1977;56(1):1–37.

[3] Belting M, Dorrell MI, Sandgren S, Aguilar E, Ahamed J, Dorfleutner A, Carmeliet P, Mueller BM, Friedlander M, Ruf W. Regulation of angiogenesis by tissue factor cytoplasmic domain signaling. Nat Med 2004;10(5):502–9.

[4] Ruf W, Mueller BM. Thrombin generation and the pathogenesis of cancer. Semin Thromb Hemost 2006;32(Suppl. 1):61–8.

[5] Angelillo-Scherrer A. Leukocyte-derived microparticles in vascular homeostasis. Circ Res 2012;110(2):356–69.

[6] Leroyer AS, Anfosso F, Lacroix R, Sabatier F, Simoncini S, Njock SM, Jourde N, Brunet P, Camoin-Jau L, Sampol J, Dignat-George F. Endothelial-derived microparticles: biological conveyors at the crossroad of inflammation, thrombosis and angiogenesis. Thromb Haemost 2010;104(3):456–63.

[7] Rautou PE, Vion AC, Amabile N, Chironi G, Simon A, Tedgui A, Boulanger CM. Microparticles, vascular function, and atherothrombosis. Circ Res 2011;109(5):593–606.

[8] Pawlinski R, Pedersen B, Erlich J, Mackman N. Role of tissue factor in haemostasis, thrombosis, angiogenesis and inflammation: lessons from low tissue factor mice. Thromb Haemost 2004;92(3):444–50.

[9] Chu AJ. Tissue factor blood coagulation, and beyond: an overview. Int J Inflam 2011;2011:367284.

[10] Langer F, Bokemeyer C. Crosstalk between cancer and haemostasis. Implications for cancer biology and cancer-associated thrombosis with focus on tissue factor. Hamostaseologie 2012;32(2):95–104.

[11] Mody RS, Carson SD. Tissue factor cytoplasmic domain peptide is multiply phosphorylated in vitro. Biochemistry 1997;36(25):7869–75.

[12] Furie B, Furie BC. Mechanisms of thrombus formation. N Engl J Med 2008;359(9):938–49.

[13] Nemerson Y. Tissue factor hemostasis. Blood 1988;71(1):1–8.

[14] Paborsky LR, Caras IW, Fisher KL, Gorman CM. Lipid association, but not the transmembrane domain, is required for tissue factor activity. Substitution of the transmembrane domain with a phosphatidylinositol anchor. J Biol Chem 1991;266(32):21911–6.

[15] Bazan JF. Structural design and molecular evolution of a cytokine receptor superfamily. Proc Natl Acad Sci USA 1990;87(18):6934–8.

[16] Chu AJ. Tissue factor mediates inflammation. Arch Biochem Biophys 2005;440(2):123–32.

[17] Bukowska A, Zacharias I, Weinert S, Skopp K, Hartmann C, Huth C, Goette A. Coagulation factor Xa induces an inflammatory signalling by activation of protease-activated receptors in human atrial tissue. Eur J Pharmacol 2013;718(1–3):114–23.

[18] Ruf W. Tissue factor and cancer. Thromb Res 2012;130(Suppl. 1):S84–7.

[19] Schaffner F, Yokota N, Ruf W. Tissue factor proangiogenic signaling in cancer progression. Thromb Res 2012;129(Suppl. 1):S127–31.

[20] Coughlin SR. Thrombin signalling protease-activated receptors. Nature 2000;407(6801):258–64.

[21] Bohm SK, Kong W, Bromme D, Smeekens SP, Anderson DC, Connolly A, Kahn M, Nelken NA, Coughlin SR, Payan DG, Bunnett NW. Molecular cloning, expression and potential functions of the human proteinase-activated receptor-2. Biochem J 1996;314(Pt. 3):1009–16.

[22] Camerer E, Huang W, Coughlin SR. Tissue factor- and factor X-dependent activation of protease-activated receptor 2 by factor VIIa. Proc Natl Acad Sci USA 2000;97(10):5255–60.

[23] Even-Ram S, Uziely B, Cohen P, Grisaru-Granovsky S, Maoz M, Ginzburg Y, Reich R, Vlodavsky I, Bar-Shavit R. Thrombin receptor overexpression in malignant and physiological invasion processes. Nat Med 1998;4(8):909–14.

[24] Even-Ram SC, Maoz M, Pokroy E, Reich R, Katz BZ, Gutwein P, Altevogt P, Bar-Shavit R. Tumor cell invasion is promoted by activation of protease activated receptor-1 in cooperation with the $\alpha v \beta 5$ integrin. J Biol Chem 2001;276(14):10952–62.

[25] Henrikson KP, Salazar SL, Fenton JW. 2nd Pentecost BT. Role of thrombin receptor in breast cancer invasiveness. Br J Cancer 1999;79(3–4): 401–6.

[26] Miyata S, Koshikawa N, Yasumitsu H, Miyazaki K. Trypsin stimulates integrin $\alpha 5 \beta 1$-dependent adhesion to fibronectin and proliferation of human gastric carcinoma cells through activation of proteinase-activated receptor-2. J Biol Chem 2000;275(7):4592–8.

[27] Nierodzik ML, Bain RM, Liu LX, Shivji M, Takeshita K, Karpatkin S. Presence of the seven transmembrane thrombin receptor on human tumour cells: effect of activation on tumour adhesion to platelets and tumor tyrosine phosphorylation. Br J Haematol 1996;92(2):452–7.

[28] Okamoto T, Nishibori M, Sawada K, Iwagaki H, Nakaya N, Jikuhara A, Tanaka N, Saeki K. The effects of stimulating protease-activated receptor-1 and -2 in A172 human glioblastoma. J Neural Transm (Vienna) 2001;108(2):125–40.

[29] Wojtukiewicz MZ, Tang DG, Ben-Josef E, Renaud C, Walz DA, Honn KV. Solid tumor cells express functional "tethered ligand" thrombin receptor. Cancer Res 1995;55(3):698–704.

[30] Riewald M, Kravchenko VV, Petrovan RJ, O'Brien PJ, Brass LF, Ulevitch RJ, Ruf W. Gene induction by coagulation factor Xa is mediated by activation of protease-activated receptor 1. Blood 2001;97(10):3109–16.

[31] Camerer E, Kataoka H, Kahn M, Lease K, Coughlin SR. Genetic evidence that protease-activated receptors mediate factor Xa signaling in endothelial cells. J Biol Chem 2002;277(18):16081–7.

[32] Pendurthi UR, Ngyuen M, Andrade-Gordon P, Petersen LC, Rao LV. Plasmin induces Cyr61 gene expression in fibroblasts via protease-activated receptor-1 and p44/42 mitogen-activated protein kinase-dependent signaling pathway. Arterioscler Thromb Vasc Biol 2002;22(9):1421–6.

[33] Majumdar M, Tarui T, Shi B, Akakura N, Ruf W, Takada Y. Plasmin-induced migration requires signaling through protease-activated receptor 1 and integrin $\alpha9\beta1$. J Biol Chem 2004;279(36):37528–34.

[34] Riewald M, Petrovan RJ, Donner A, Mueller BM, Ruf W. Activation of endothelial cell protease activated receptor 1 by the protein C pathway. Science 2002;296(5574):1880–2.

[35] Beaulieu LM, Church FC. Activated protein C promotes breast cancer cell migration through interactions with EPCR and PAR-1. Exp Cell Res 2007;313(4):677–87.

[36] Oikonomopoulou K, Hansen KK, Saifeddine M, Tea I, Blaber M, Blaber SI, Scarisbrick I, Andrade-Gordon P, Cottrell GS, Bunnett NW, Diamandis EP, Hollenberg MD. Proteinase-activated receptors, targets for kallikrein signaling. J Biol Chem 2006;281(43):32095–112.

[37] Oikonomopoulou K, Hansen KK, Saifeddine M, Vergnolle N, Tea I, Blaber M, Blaber SI, Scarisbrick I, Diamandis EP, Hollenberg MD. Kallikrein-mediated cell signalling: targeting proteinase-activated receptors (PARs). Biol Chem 2006;387(6):817–24.

[38] Boire A, Covic L, Agarwal A, Jacques S, Sherifi S, Kuliopulos A. PAR1 is a matrix metalloprotease-1 receptor that promotes invasion and tumorigenesis of breast cancer cells. Cell 2005;120(3):303–13.

[39] Riewald M, Ruf W. Mechanistic coupling of protease signaling and initiation of coagulation by tissue factor. Proc Natl Acad Sci USA 2001;98(14):7742–7.

[40] Briot A, Deraison C, Lacroix M, Bonnart C, Robin A, Besson C, Dubus P, Hovnanian A. Kallikrein 5 induces atopic dermatitis-like lesions through PAR2-mediated thymic stromal lymphopoietin expression in Netherton syndrome. J Exp Med 2009;206(5):1135–47.

[41] Frateschi S, Camerer E, Crisante G, Rieser S, Membrez M, Charles RP, Beermann F, Stehle JC, Breiden B, Sandhoff K, Rotman S, Haftek M, Wilson A, Ryser S, Steinhoff M, Coughlin SR, Hummler E. PAR2 absence completely rescues inflammation and ichthyosis caused by altered CAP1/Prss8 expression in mouse skin. Nat Commun 2011;2:161.

[42] Camerer E, Barker A, Duong DN, Ganesan R, Kataoka H, Cornelissen I, Darragh MR, Hussain A, Zheng YW, Srinivasan Y, Brown C, Xu SM, Regard JB, Lin CY, Craik CS, Kirchhofer D, Coughlin SR. Local protease signaling contributes to neural tube closure in the mouse embryo. Dev Cell 2010;18(1):25–38.

[43] Takeuchi T, Harris JL, Huang W, Yan KW, Coughlin SR, Craik CS. Cellular localization of membrane-type serine protease 1 and identification of protease-activated receptor-2 and single-chain urokinase-type plasminogen activator as substrates. J Biol Chem 2000;275(34):26333–42.

[44] Hembrough TA, Swartz GM, Papathanassiu A, Vlasuk GP, Rote WE, Green SJ, Pribluda VS. Tissue factor/factor VIIa inhibitors block angiogenesis and tumor growth through a nonhemostatic mechanism. Cancer Res 2003;63(11):2997–3000.

[45] Mousa SA. Anticoagulants in thrombosis and cancer: the missing link. Semin Thromb Hemost 2002;28(1):45–52.

[46] Mousa SA, Mohamed S. Inhibition of endothelial cell tube formation by the low molecular weight heparin, tinzaparin, is mediated by tissue factor pathway inhibitor. Thromb Haemost 2004;92(3):627–33.

[47] Mousa SA, Mohamed S. Anti-angiogenic mechanisms and efficacy of the low molecular weight heparin, tinzaparin: anti-cancer efficacy. Oncol Rep 2004;12(4):683–8.

[48] Ge L, Shenoy SK, Lefkowitz RJ, DeFea K. Constitutive protease-activated receptor-2-mediated migration of MDA MB-231 breast cancer cells requires both β-arrestin-1 and -2. J Biol Chem 2004;279(53):55419–24.

[49] Zoudilova M, Kumar P, Ge L, Wang P, Bokoch GM, DeFea KA. β-arrestin-dependent regulation of the cofilin pathway downstream of protease-activated receptor-2. J Biol Chem 2007;282(28):20634–46.

[50] Albrektsen T, Sorensen BB, Hjorto GM, Fleckner J, Rao LV, Petersen LC. Transcriptional program induced by factor VIIa-tissue factor, PAR1 and PAR2 in MDA-MB-231 cells. J Thromb Haemost 2007;5(8):1588–97.

[51] Ahamed J, Ruf W. Protease-activated receptor 2-dependent phosphorylation of the tissue factor cytoplasmic domain. J Biol Chem 2004;279(22):23038–44.

[52] Dorfleutner A, Ruf W. Regulation of tissue factor cytoplasmic domain phosphorylation by palmitoylation. Blood 2003;102(12):3998–4005.

[53] Sorensen BB, Freskgard PO, Nielsen LS, Rao LV, Ezban M, Petersen LC. Factor VIIa-induced p44/42 mitogen-activated protein kinase activation requires the proteolytic activity of factor VIIa and is independent of the tissue factor cytoplasmic domain. J Biol Chem 1999;274(30):21349–54.

[54] Versteeg HH, Hoedemaeker I, Diks SH, Stam JC, Spaargaren M. van Bergen En Henegouwen PM, van Deventer SJ, Peppelenbosch MP. Factor VIIa/tissue factor-induced signaling via activation of Src-like kinases, phosphatidylinositol 3-kinase, and Rac. J Biol Chem 2000;275(37):28750–6.

[55] Versteeg HH, Peppelenbosch MP, Spek CA. The pleiotropic effects of tissue factor: a possible role for factor VIIa-induced intracellular signalling? Thromb Haemost 2001;86(6):1353–9.

[56] Camerer E, Rottingen JA, Gjernes E, Larsen K, Skartlien AH, Iversen JG, Prydz H. Coagulation factors VIIa and Xa induce cell signaling leading to up-regulation of the *egr*-1 gene. J Biol Chem 1999;274(45):32225–33.

[57] Zucker S, Mirza H, Conner CE, Lorenz AF, Drews MH, Bahou WF, Jesty J. Vascular endothelial growth factor induces tissue factor and matrix metalloproteinase production in endothelial cells: conversion of prothrombin to thrombin results in progelatinase A activation and cell proliferation. Int J Cancer 1998;75(5):780–6.

[58] Woods SA, McGlade CJ, Guha A. Phosphatidylinositol 3'-kinase and MAPK/ERK kinase 1/2 differentially regulate expression of vascular endothelial growth factor in human malignant astrocytoma cells. Neuro Oncol 2002;4(4):242–52.

[59] Jung YD, Liu W, Reinmuth N, Ahmad SA, Fan F, Gallick GE, Ellis LM. Vascular endothelial growth factor is upregulated by interleukin-1 β in human vascular smooth muscle cells via the P38 mitogen-activated protein kinase pathway. Angiogenesis 2001;4(2):155–62.

[60] Tsai PW, Shiah SG, Lin MT, Wu CW, Kuo ML. Up-regulation of vascular endothelial growth factor C in breast cancer cells by heregulin-β 1. A critical role of p38/nuclear factor-κ B signaling pathway. J Biol Chem 2003;278(8):5750–9.

[61] Hoshi S, Nomoto K, Kuromitsu J, Tomari S, Nagata M. High glucose induced VEGF expression via PKC and ERK in glomerular podocytes. Biochem Biophys Res Commun 2002;290(1):177–84.

[62] Xu L, Fukumura D, Jain RK. Acidic extracellular pH induces vascular endothelial growth factor (VEGF) in human glioblastoma cells via ERK1/2 MAPK signaling pathway: mechanism of low pH-induced VEGF. J Biol Chem 2002;277(13):11368–74.

[63] Maity A, Pore N, Lee J, Solomon D, O'Rourke DM. Epidermal growth factor receptor transcriptionally up-regulates vascular endothelial growth

factor expression in human glioblastoma cells via a pathway involving phosphatidylinositol 3'-kinase and distinct from that induced by hypoxia. Cancer Res 2000;60(20):5879–86.

[64] Mori K, Tani M, Kamata K, Kawamura H, Urata Y, Goto S, Kuwano M, Shibata S, Kondo T. Mitogen-activated protein kinase, ERK1/2, is essential for the induction of vascular endothelial growth factor by ionizing radiation mediated by activator protein-1 in human glioblastoma cells. Free Radic Res 2000;33(2):157–66.

[65] Suzuma I, Suzuma K, Ueki K, Hata Y, Feener EP, King GL, Aiello LP. Stretch-induced retinal vascular endothelial growth factor expression is mediated by phosphatidylinositol 3-kinase and protein kinase C (PKC)-zeta but not by stretch-induced ERK1/2, Akt, Ras, or classical/novel PKC pathways. J Biol Chem 2002;277(2):1047–57.

[66] Pai R, Szabo IL, Soreghan BA, Atay S, Kawanaka H, Tarnawski AS. PGE(2) stimulates VEGF expression in endothelial cells via ERK2/JNK1 signaling pathways. Biochem Biophys Res Commun 2001;286(5):923–8.

[67] Berra E, Pages G, Pouyssegur J. MAP kinases and hypoxia in the control of VEGF expression. Cancer Metastasis Rev 2000;19(1-2):139–45.

[68] Berra E, Milanini J, Richard DE, Le Gall M, Vinals F, Gothie E, Roux D, Pages G, Pouyssegur J. Signaling angiogenesis via p42/p44 MAP kinase and hypoxia. Biochem Pharmacol 2000;60(8):1171–8.

[69] Jung YD, Nakano K, Liu W, Gallick GE, Ellis LM. Extracellular signal-regulated kinase activation is required for up-regulation of vascular endothelial growth factor by serum starvation in human colon carcinoma cells. Cancer Res 1999;59(19):4804–7.

[70] Stojkovic S, Kaun C, Basilio J, Rauscher S, Hell L, Krychtiuk KA, Bonstingl C, de Martin R, Groger M, Ay C, Holnthoner W, Eppel W, Neumayer C, Huk I, Huber K, Demyanets S, Wojta J. Tissue factor is induced by interleukin-33 in human endothelial cells: a new link between coagulation and inflammation. Sci Rep 2016;6:25171.

[71] Choi YS, Choi HJ, Min JK, Pyun BJ, Maeng YS, Park H, Kim J, Kim YM, Kwon YG. Interleukin-33 induces angiogenesis and vascular permeability through ST2/TRAF6-mediated endothelial nitric oxide production. Blood 2009;114(14):3117–26.

[72] Demetz G, Seitz I, Stein A, Steppich B, Groha P, Brandl R, Schomig A, Ott I. Tissue Factor-Factor VIIa complex induces cytokine expression in coronary artery smooth muscle cells. Atherosclerosis 2010;212(2):466–71.

[73] Virchow R. Die krankhaften Geschwulste. Berlin: Hirschwald; 1863.

[74] Balkwill F, Mantovani A. Inflammation and cancer: back to Virchow? Lancet 2001;357(9255):539–45.

[75] Koong AC, Denko NC, Hudson KM, Schindler C, Swiersz L, Koch C, Evans S, Ibrahim H, Le QT, Terris DJ, Giaccia AJ. Candidate genes for the hypoxic tumor phenotype. Cancer Res 2000;60(4):883–7.

[76] Rong Y, Post DE, Pieper RO, Durden DL, Van Meir EG, Brat DJ. PTEN and hypoxia regulate tissue factor expression and plasma coagulation by glioblastoma. Cancer Res 2005;65(4):1406–13.

[77] Naldini A, Sower L, Bocci V, Meyers B, Carney DH. Thrombin receptor expression and responsiveness of human monocytic cells to thrombin is linked to interferon-induced cellular differentiation. J Cell Physiol 1998;177(1):76–84.

[78] McLean K, Schirm S, Johns A, Morser J, Light DR. FXa-induced responses in vascular wall cells are PAR-mediated and inhibited by ZK-807834. Thromb Res 2001;103(4):281–97.

[79] Jones A, Geczy CL. Thrombin and factor Xa enhance the production of interleukin-1. Immunology 1990;71(2):236–41.

[80] Senden NH, Jeunhomme TM, Heemskerk JW, Wagenvoord R, van't Veer C, Hemker HC, Buurman WA. Factor Xa induces cytokine production and expression of adhesion molecules by human umbilical vein endothelial cells. J Immunol 1998;161(8):4318–24.

[81] Ollivier V, Chabbat J, Herbert JM, Hakim J, de Prost D. Vascular endothelial growth factor production by fibroblasts in response to factor VIIa binding to tissue factor involves thrombin and factor Xa. Arterioscler Thromb Vasc Biol 2000;20(5):1374–81.

[82] Bar D, Apte RN, Voronov E, Dinarello CA, Cohen S. A continuous delivery system of IL-1 receptor antagonist reduces angiogenesis and inhibits tumor development. FASEB J 2004;18(1):161–3.

[83] Voronov E, Carmi Y, Apte RN. Role of IL-1-mediated inflammation in tumor angiogenesis. Adv Exp Med Biol 2007;601:265–70.

[84] Voronov E, Carmi Y, Apte RN. The role IL-1 in tumor-mediated angiogenesis. Front Physiol 2014;5:114.

[85] Botto S, Streblow DN, DeFilippis V, White L, Kreklywich CN, Smith PP, Caposio P. IL-6 in human cytomegalovirus secretome promotes angiogenesis and survival of endothelial cells through the stimulation of survivin. Blood 2011;117(1):352–61.

[86] Liu Q, Li G, Li R, Shen J, He Q, Deng L, Zhang C, Zhang J. IL-6 promotion of glioblastoma cell invasion and angiogenesis in U251 and T98G cell lines. J Neurooncol 2010;100(2):165–76.

[87] Liu X, Liu K, Qin J, Hao L, Li X, Liu Y, Zhang X, Liu X, Li P, Han S, Mao Z, Shen L. C/EBPβ promotes angiogenesis through secretion of IL-6, which is inhibited by genistein, in EGFRvIII-positive glioblastoma. Int J Cancer 2015;136(11):2524–34.

[88] Niu J, Azfer A, Zhelyabovska O, Fatma S, Kolattukudy PE. Monocyte chemotactic protein (MCP)-1 promotes angiogenesis via a novel transcription factor MCP-1-induced protein (MCPIP). J Biol Chem 2008;283(21):14542–51.

[89] Salcedo R, Ponce ML, Young HA, Wasserman K, Ward JM, Kleinman HK, Oppenheim JJ, Murphy WJ. Human endothelial cells express CCR2 and respond to MCP-1: direct role of MCP-1 in angiogenesis and tumor progression. Blood 2000;96(1):34–40.

[90] Goede V, Brogelli L, Ziche M, Augustin HG. Induction of inflammatory angiogenesis by monocyte chemoattractant protein-1. Int J Cancer 1999;82(5):765–70.

[91] Costa C, Incio J, Soares R. Angiogenesis. Angiogenesis and chronic inflammation: cause or consequence? 2007;10(3):149–66.

[92] Cunningham MA, Romas P, Hutchinson P, Holdsworth SR, Tipping PG. Tissue factor and factor VIIa receptor/ligand interactions induce proinflammatory effects in macrophages. Blood 1999;94(10):3413–20.

[93] Camerer E, Rottingen JA, Iversen JG, Prydz H. Coagulation factors VII and X induce Ca^{2+} oscillations in Madin-Darby canine kidney cells only when proteolytically active. J Biol Chem 1996;271(46):29034–42.

[94] Poulsen LK, Jacobsen N, Sorensen BB, Bergenhem NC, Kelly JD, Foster DC, Thastrup O, Ezban M, Petersen LC. Signal transduction via the mitogen-activated protein kinase pathway induced by binding of coagulation factor VIIa to tissue factor. J Biol Chem 1998;273(11):6228–32.

[95] Pendurthi UR, Alok D, Rao LV. Proc Natl Acad Sci USA. Binding of factor VIIa to tissue factor induces alterations in gene expression in human fibroblast cells: up-regulation of poly(A) polymerase 1997;94(23): 12598–603.

[96] Taniguchi T, Kakkar AK, Tuddenham EG, Williamson RC, Lemoine NR. Enhanced expression of urokinase receptor induced through the tissue factor-factor VIIa pathway in human pancreatic cancer. Cancer Res 1998;58(19):4461–7.

[97] Siegbahn A, Johnell M, Rorsman C, Ezban M, Heldin CH, Ronnstrand L. Binding of factor VIIa to tissue factor on human fibroblasts leads to activation of phospholipase C and enhanced PDGF-BB-stimulated chemotaxis. Blood 2000;96(10):3452–8.

[98] Pendurthi UR, Allen KE, Ezban M, Rao LV. Factor VIIa and thrombin induce the expression of Cyr61 and connective tissue growth factor, extracellular matrix signaling proteins that could act as possible downstream mediators in factor VIIa · tissue factor-induced signal transduction. J Biol Chem 2000;275(19):14632–41.

CHAPTER 5

microRNAs and Angiogenesis

Paul J. Davis, Matthew Leinung and Shaker A. Mousa

Contents

INTRODUCTION

microRNAs (miRs, miRNAs) are a category of small, single-stranded, noncoding RNAs, 18–25 nucleotides in length, that bind to specific messenger RNAs (mRNAs) to regulate gene expression. They are evolutionarily well-conserved. miRs represent fewer than 2% of all of the genes of mammals, but this may amount to 30% or more of protein-coding genes [1–6]. As of 2015, the existence of more than 1200 human miRNAs has been validated [7,8]. miRNAs affect expression of their target mRNAs via their content of specific sequences that are complimentary to those of specific mRNAs [9–11]. Binding by a target mRNA of a specific miRNA may result in the decay of the mRNA or in inhibition of translation of the mRNA [12].

One miRNA may recognize and target a hundred or several hundred different mRNAs. Thus, interpretation of the results of a given miRNA study does not permit systematic construction of the molecular mechanism by which an end result, for example, the down- or upregulation of vascular endothelial growth factor (*VEGF*) gene expression, is achieved. Much of the activity of

Anti-Angiogenesis Strategies in Cancer Therapies
http://dx.doi.org/10.1016/B978-0-12-802576-5.00005-X

miRNAs is directed at components of signal transduction pathways critical to the expression of genes, or for action of the gene products, involved in blood vessel manipulation.

A substantial number of miRNAs are implicated in the regulation of angiogenesis via effects on VEGF (Table 5.1). The end result of altered protein abundance may include a *direct* anti-translational miRNA effect on cytoplasmic *VEGF* mRNA; however, it is clear that most of the effects of the miRNA(s) of interest may be inserted upstream in the complex signal transduction mechanism of control of VEGF production by the mRNAs of angiogenesis-relevant and VEGF-relevant intermediary signaling factors. Examples of the latter are the mRNAs of p70S6K1 [13,14], p120RasGAP [15], phosphatidylinositol 3-phosphate kinase (PI3-K/PTEN/Akt) [16], and other targets of angiogenesis-linked miRNAs that culminate in actions on VEGF mRNAs, often through hypoxia-inducible factor-1α (HIF-1α). p120RasGAP (Ras GTPase-activating protein) serves as a molecular brake for Ras [15], maintaining endothelial cells in a quiescent state; downregulation of p120RasGAP and Ras is a component of the proangiogenic "switch" by which new blood vessel formation is turned on. It has been pointed out that the off-on switch characterization of the regulation of angiogenesis by miRNAs may instead be a "fine-tuning" process [17]. A downstream target of MTOR (mammalian target of rapamycin), p70S6K1 (serine/threonine protein kinase 1) contributes to the control of tumor cell cycle and proliferation as well as regulation of expression of HIF-1α and VEGF genes. Specific miRNAs, such as these that have been shown in vivo to be heavily committed to regulation of angiogenesis have been termed angiomiRs [18,19].

miRNAs are in large measure encoded in the introns of genes or intergenic regions of DNA and generated via RNA polymerase III as primary transcripts. Nuclear transcription factors contribute to the transcript generation. The transcripts are cleaved by double-strand RNA proteins, for example, Drosha [17], resulting in a 55–70 nucleotide hairpin RNA that is released by specific factors, for example, Exportin-5, from the nucleus [5]. Mature 22-nucleotide

Table 5.1 Angiogenesis-relevant microRNAs (miR)

Action	miR	Mechanism; intermediate target messenger RNAs (mRNAs)	References
Proangiogenesis			
	miR–126	Modulate endothelial cell response to VEGF	[20,21]
	miR–27b	Endothelial cell activation	[22]
	miR–93	Enhance endothelial cell proliferation; p21, E2F1	[23]
	miR–210	Enhance endothelial cell migration, formation of capillaries	[24]
	miR–378a	Enhance angiogenesis; Fus–1	[25,26]
		VEGF; SHH	[27]
	miR–296	Increase abundance of proangiogenic growth factor receptors	[28]
	miR–10b	Regulate endothelial cell division, migration	[29]
	miR–196b	Unknown	[30]
	miR–130a	Suppress anti-angiogenic gene transcription	[31]
	miR–132	Increase Ras activity; Activate endothelial cells	[32]
	miR–497/VEGF–A	Increase tube formation; Twist	[33]
Anti-angiogenesis			
	miR–519c	Decrease tube-formation; HIF–1α	[34]
	miR–214	Decrease sprouting; QK1	[35]
	miR–200 family	Decrease angiogenesis via IL–8, CXCL1	[36,37]
	miR–107	Hypoxia signaling	[38]
	miR–15a	Control of angiogenesis, cell proliferation; VEGF–A	[39]
	miR–16	VEGF expression	[39,40]
	miR–199a	Interference with tumor-related angiogenesis (VEGF, HIF–1α)	[41]
	miR–125b	Depress cancer-related angiogenesis via HIF–1α/VEGF	[41]
	miR–361–5p	Depress cancer-related angiogenesis via VEGF–A	[42]

(Continued)

Table 5.1 Angiogenesis-relevant microRNAs (miR) (cont.)

Action	miR	Mechanism; intermediate target messenger RNAs (mRNAs)	References
	miR–1/206	Downregulate VEGF-A	[43]
	miR–503	Depress cancer-related angiogenesis via VEGF-A, FGF2	[44]
	miR–128	Depress cancer-related angiogenesis via p70S6K1	[13]
	miR–145	Depress cancer-related angiogenesis via p70S6K1	[14]
	miR–26a	Depress cancer-related angiogenesis via HIF-1α, Akt; cMet	[16,45]
	miR–34 family	Cardiac remodeling; VEGF, Notch1	[46]
	miR–26b-5p	Decrease microvessel density; VE-cadherin; MMP2	[47]
	miR–218	Decrease retinal neovascularization; Robo1	[48]
	miR–137	Decrease angiogenesis; NUCKS1	[49]
	miR–195a-3p	Decrease choroidal neovascularization; MMP2	[50]
	miR–17-92	Decrease tumor angiogenesis; HIF-1α, VEGF-A	[51]
	miR–124	AKT2	[52]
Proangiogenesis, anti-angiogenesis	miR–221/222	Inhibit SCF	[53–55]
	miR–424	Destabilize E3-ligase assembly via VEGF, VEGFR–2, FGFR–1	[40,56]
	miR–21	Proangiogenesis: Increase tube formation; TIMP3, MMPs, HIF-1α, VEGF	[57,58]
		Anti-angiogenesis: Resistance to hypoxia, inhibition of tumor-related angiogenesis	[59–61]

Abbreviations: Akt, Protein kinase B (PKB); AKT2, AKT serine/threonine kinase 2; cMet, hepatocyte growth factor receptor; CXCL1, chemokine (C–X–C motif) ligand 1; FGF fibroblast growth factor; FGFR fibroblast growth factor receptor; Fus–1, nuclear fusion protein Fus–1; HIF–1α, hypoxia-inducible factor–1 alpha; IL–8, interleukin–8; MMP, matrix metalloproteinase; NUCKS, nuclear casein kinase; p70S6K1, p70S6 kinase (a serine/threonine kinase); QK1, Quaking; SCF, stem cell factor; SHH, sonic hedgehog; TIMP3 metalloproteinase inhibitor 3; Robo1, roundabout homolog 1; VEGF, vascular endothelial growth factor; VEGFR, vascular endothelial growth factor receptor.

duplex RNAs are generated in cytoplasm from the 55–70 nucleotide pre-miRs by an RNA III enzyme, Dicer [17,62]. Dicer is essential to the elaboration of large numbers of miRs. The genetic disabling of Dicer and consequent disordering of angiogenesis in mouse embryos was an initial step in establishing the important contributions of miRNAs to angiogenesis [63].

The cytoplasmic domain of miRNAs is complimented by their packaging in exosomes [64]. These up to 100 nm diameter vesicles may have specific profiles of miRNA content and, after cellular release, may be taken up by adjacent cells or distant cells following exosomal entry into the circulation. The miRNA-containing exosome can alter the phenotype of recipient cells, but it is not yet clear whether the packaging of miRNAs in these vesicles is random or directed by an organized process within the originating cell.

SPECIFIC miRNAs AND ANGIOGENESIS

Following the studies of disordered angiogenesis that resulted from specific deletion of Dicer in several models [63,65,66], the definition of roles of specific miRNAs began with studies of miR-221/222 [53] and of the most abundant miR in endothelial cells, miR-126 [20,21,67,68].

Anand and coworkers [32] and others [69–71] demonstrated the importance of miR-132 to proper function of endothelial and vascular smooth muscle cells. In a subsequent review, Anand [5] listed 10 miRs that were felt to be of particular relevance to blood vessel formation. These miRs included the Let-7 family (endothelial cell proliferation), miR-126 (amplification in endothelial cells of the effects of VEGF), miR-132 (amplified growth factor signaling), miR-210 (genesis of vascular tubes), miR-221/222 (inhibition of angiogenesis), miR-296 (inhibition of growth factor receptor recycling), miR-424 (stabilization of hypoxia-induced factor-1), miR-92a (inhibition of angiogenesis), miR-143-145 (support of differentiation of vascular smooth muscle cells), and miR–26a (support of vascular smooth muscle cell proliferation). Fully committed to the regulation of angiogenesis, endothelial cell miR–126 is an example of an angiomiR.

A very large complement of miRNAs, in addition to those identified earlier, has now been shown to impact the angiogenic process (Table 5.1). The panel of miRNAs may be proangiogenic, anti-angiogenic, or both, depending on the set of angiogenesis-relevant mRNAs with which the miRNAs interact.

Endothelial Cells and miRNAs

miR–126 is a paradigm of a microRNA primarily involved in blood vessel formation and is the principal miRNA resident in endothelial cells, as noted above. Its activity is largely expressed via VEGF. A variety of traits of activated endothelial cells—migration in response to chemical cues, cell division, formation of primordial vessels/tube formation—are associated with miRNAs. These include, but are not limited to miR–126, miR–27b, miR–93, miR–210, miR–10b, and miR–132 (Table 5.1).

miRNAs and Hypoxia

The stimulus to angiogenesis of hypoxia has long been appreciated. It is a component of organ rescue in the heart and other tissues and may contribute to tumor aggressiveness or to tissue defense. In the case of the latter, the core of a spherical tumor may be hypoxic and relatively resistant to the angiogenic stimulation. Functionally, reduced vascular supply isolates core tumor cells from chemotherapy and host immune defenses; unrepaired hypoxia renders tumor cells relatively radioresistant, since they do not undergo cell division. Table 5.1 indicates that miR–21, miR–107, miR–125b, miR–199a, and miR–17–92 are anti-angiogenic, largely via downregulation of HIF-1α. Thus, these miRNAs are defensive. The absence of a set of miRNAs that support transcription of HIF-1α suggests that this pathway is not essential to tumor invasiveness and that angiogenesis in support of cancer aggressiveness not unexpectedly relates to miRNAs and mRNAs for vascular growth factors, chiefly VEGF, for endothelial cell activity/migration and tubular sprouting.

miRNAs and VEGF

The spectrum of pro- and anti-angiogenic miRNAs listed in Table 5.1 involves actions on vascular growth factors. As noted earlier, miR-126 stimulates VEGF signaling and expression [67,72] and, in turn, specific miRNAs may be upregulated by VEGF and basic fibroblast growth factor (bFGF) [32]. miR-126 and miR-132 can also stimulate angiogenesis indirectly by decreasing expression of negative regulators of VEGF signaling [5].

miRNAs and Hormone-Stimulated Angiogenesis

Thyroid hormone. The proangiogenic properties of thyroid hormone have been defined by a number of laboratories, beginning with a demonstration of new blood formation in the ischemic myocardium exposed to increased concentrations of L-thyroxine (T_4) [73]. Although the intracellular biological activity of thyroid hormone is due to 3,5,3'-triiodo-L-thyronine (T_3) derived from T_4 and acting at intranuclear thyroid hormone receptors (TRs), it has become clear that T_4, itself, stimulates angiogenesis. This effect is initiated at a thyroid hormone receptor on the extracellular domain of plasma membrane integrin $\alpha v \beta 3$ [74–76]. Angiogenesis stimulated by T_4 involves crosstalk between the integrin and adjacent vascular growth factor receptors and a panel of genomic effects on bFGF [77] and VEGF gene expression, endothelial cell motility [78] and matrix metalloproteinases [79].

A deaminated metabolite of T_4, tetraiodothyroacetic acid (tetrac), inhibits binding of T_4 to the receptor on $\alpha v \beta 3$ and blocks the angiogenic activity of T_4 [76,78]. This may be of particular importance to cancer-related blood vessel formation. Recently, we have shown that a nanoparticulate formulation of tetrac that acts on the integrin has selective actions on the generation of miRs. For example, the expression of miR-21, a proangiogenic, anti-apoptotic product of tumor cells, is downregulated by nanoparticulate tetrac

(Nanotetrac, Nano-diamino-tetrac, NDAT) [80]. This implies that T_4, the form of thyroid hormone whose actions at $\alpha v \beta 3$ are blocked by Nanotetrac, upregulates transcription of this factor, but this has not as yet been examined experimentally. Among the angiogenesis-relevant genes whose expression is upregulated by miR-21 are HIF-1α [81], VEGF, and Angiopoietin-1 [72]. Thus, the complex anti-angiogenic activity of tetrac formulations initiated at integrin $\alpha v \beta 3$ is likely to be in part mediated by down-regulation of miR-21; this infers that proangiogenic T_4 activity may depend in part upon expression of this miRNA.

Vitamin D. Vitamin D induces a large number of miRNAs [82], among which is miR-93 (Table 5.1). Endothelial cell proliferation supported by vitamin D results from miRNA targeting of p21 and E2F1.

Estrogen. Among the microRNAs induced by estrogen is miR-124 (miR-124/AKT2) (Table 5.1) [52]. Although estrogen is proangiogenic by multiple mechanisms, the angiogenesis-relevant miR-124 produced in response to estrogen is anti-angiogenic. The target of this miRNA is mRNA for signal transducing Akt.

Clinical Targeting of miRNAs

The practicality of clinical anti-miRNA therapy has been a matter of investigative interest for more than a decade [4]. There are multiple molecular strategies. These include locked nucleic acid (LNA) anti-miRs [83], oligonucleotides engineered to silence host miRs (antagomirs) [84], miR-masks, and miR sponges. The masks are single-stranded 2'-O-methyl anti-sense oligonucleotides exactly complementary to assumed miRNA binding regions of the 3'-untranslated regions in the mRNA of interest [85]. The sponges are miRNA-inhibiting transgenes that express mRNAs with several binding sites intended to attract target miRNAs and block the binding of the latter to endogenous (target) mRNAs [86]. There are several other approaches to anti-miRNA therapy [4].

Certain of these strategies have had encouraging preclinical anti-cancer results [87,88], and several clinical trials that target specific miRNAs relevant to cancer are in progress (https://clinicaltrials. gov/). An important issue remains the molecular caprice of specific miRs, that is, a given miRNA recognizes a cadre of mRNAs in addition to the mRNA of interest. The risk of an unfavorable side effect profile thus exists, unless it is practical to deliver a therapeutic miR to a tissue target site, such as a tumor.

REFERENCES

[1] Bartel DP. MicroRNAs: target recognition and regulatory functions. Cell 2009;136(2):215–33.

[2] Kozomara A, Griffiths-Jones S. miRBase: integrating microRNA annotation and deep-sequencing data. Nucleic Acids Res 2011;39:D152–7.

[3] Lagos-Quintana M, Rauhut R, Lendeckel W, Tuschl T. Identification of novel genes coding for small expressed RNAs. Science 2001;294(5543):853–8.

[4] Gallach S, Calabuig-Farinas S, Jantus-Lewintre E, Camps C. MicroRNAs: promising new antiangiogenic targets in cancer. BioMed Res Int 2014;2014:878450.

[5] Anand S. A brief primer on microRNAs and their roles in angiogenesis. Vasc Cell 2013;5(1):2.

[6] Krol J, Loedige I, Filipowicz W. The widespread regulation of microRNA biogenesis, function and decay. Nat Rev Genet 2010;11(9):597–610.

[7] MacDonagh L, Gray SG, Finn SP, Cuffe S, O'Byrne KJ, Barr MP. The emerging role of microRNAs in resistance to lung cancer treatments. Cancer Treat Rev 2015;41(2):160–9.

[8] Lee RC, Feinbaum RL, Ambros V. The *C. elegans* heterochronic gene lin-4 encodes small RNAs with antisense complementarity to lin-14. Cell 1993;75(5):843–54.

[9] Esquela-Kerscher A, Slack FJ. Oncomirs—microRNAs with a role in cancer. Nat Rev Cancer 2006;6(4):259–69.

[10] Meltzer PS. Cancer genomics: small RNAs with big impacts. Nature 2005;435(7043):745–6.

[11] Garzon R, Fabbri M, Cimmino A, Calin GA, Croce CM. MicroRNA expression and function in cancer. Trends Mol Med 2006;12(12):580–7.

[12] Carthew RW, Sontheimer EJ. Origins and mechanisms of miRNAs and siRNAs. Cell 2009;136(4):642–55.

[13] Shi ZM, Wang J, Yan Z, You YP, Li CY, Qian X, Yin Y, Zhao P, Wang YY, Wang XF, Li MN, Liu LZ, Liu N, Jiang BH. MiR-128 inhibits tumor growth and angiogenesis by targeting p70S6K1. PLoS One 2012;7(3):e32709.

[14] Xu Q, Liu LZ, Qian X, Chen Q, Jiang Y, Li D, Lai L, Jiang BH. MiR-145 directly targets p70S6K1 in cancer cells to inhibit tumor growth and angiogenesis. Nucleic Acids Res 2012;40(2):761–74.

[15] Anand S, Cheresh DA. MicroRNA-mediated regulation of the angiogenic switch. Curr Opin Hematol 2011;18(3):171–6.

[16] Chai ZT, Kong J, Zhu XD, Zhang YY, Lu L, Zhou JM, Wang LR, Zhang KZ, Zhang QB, Ao JY, Wang M, Wu WZ, Wang L, Tang ZY, Sun HC. MicroRNA-26a inhibits angiogenesis by down-regulating VEGFA through the PIK3C2α/Akt/HIF-1α pathway in hepatocellular carcinoma. PLoS One 2013;8(10):e77957.

[17] Landskroner-Eiger S, Moneke I, Sessa WC. miRNAs as modulators of angiogenesis. Cold Spring Harb Perspect Med 2013;3(2):a006643.

[18] Wang SS, Olson EN. AngiomiRs-Key regulators of angiogenesis. Curr Opin Genet Dev 2009;19(3):205–11.

[19] Matejuk A, Collet G, Nadim M, Grillon C, Kieda C. MicroRNAs and tumor vasculature normalization: impact on anti-tumor immune response. Arch Immunol Ther Exp (Warsz) 2013;61(4):285–99.

[20] Fish JE, Santoro MM, Morton SU, Yu S, Yeh RF, Wythe JD, Ivey KN, Bruneau BG, Stainier DY, Srivastava D. miR-126 regulates angiogenic signaling and vascular integrity. Dev Cell 2008;15(2):272–84.

[21] Wang S, Aurora AB, Johnson BA, Qi X, McAnally J, Hill JA, Richardson JA, Bassel-Duby R, Olson EN. The endothelial-specific microRNA miR-126 governs vascular integrity and angiogenesis. Dev Cell 2008;15(2):261–71.

[22] Suarez Y, Sessa WC. MicroRNAs as novel regulators of angiogenesis. Circ Res 2009;104(4):442–54.

[23] Fang L, Du WW, Yang W, Rutnam ZJ, Peng C, Li H, O'Malley YQ, Askeland RW, Sugg S, Liu M, Mehta T, Deng Z, Yang BB. MiR-93 enhances angiogenesis and metastasis by targeting LATS2. Cell Cycle 2012;11(23):4352–65.

[24] Fasanaro P, D'Alessandra Y, Di Stefano V, Melchionna R, Romani S, Pompilio G, Capogrossi MC, Martelli F. MicroRNA-210 modulates endothelial cell response to hypoxia and inhibits the receptor tyrosine kinase ligand Ephrin-A3. J Biol Chem 2008;283(23):15878–83.

[25] Hua Z, Lv Q, Ye W, Wong CK, Cai G, Gu D, Ji Y, Zhao C, Wang J, Yang BB, Zhang Y. MiRNA-directed regulation of VEGF and other angiogenic factors under hypoxia. PLoS One 2006;1:e116.

[26] Lee DY, Deng Z, Wang CH, Yang BB. MicroRNA-378 promotes cell survival, tumor growth, and angiogenesis by targeting SuFu and Fus-1 expression. Proc Natl Acad Sci USA 2007;104(51):20350–30255.

[27] Krist B, Florczyk U, Pietraszek-Gremplewicz K, Jozkowicz A, Dulak J. The role of miR-378a in metabolism, angiogenesis, and muscle biology. Int J Endocrinol 2015;2015:281756.

[28] Wurdinger T, Tannous BA, Saydam O, Skog J, Grau S, Soutschek J, Weissleder R, Breakefield XO, Krichevsky AM. miR-296 regulates growth factor receptor overexpression in angiogenic endothelial cells. Cancer Cell 2008;14(5):382–93.

[29] Hassel D, Cheng P, White MP, Ivey KN, Kroll J, Augustin HG, Katus HA, Stainier DY, Srivastava D. MicroRNA-10 regulates the angiogenic behavior of zebrafish and human endothelial cells by promoting vascular endothelial growth factor signaling. Circ Res 2012;111(11):1421–33.

[30] Plummer PN, Freeman R, Taft RJ, Vider J, Sax M, Umer BA, Gao D, Johns C, Mattick JS, Wilton SD, Ferro V, McMillan NA, Swarbrick A, Mittal V, Mellick AS. MicroRNAs regulate tumor angiogenesis modulated by endothelial progenitor cells. Cancer Res 2013;73(1):341–52.

[31] Chen Y, Gorski DH. Regulation of angiogenesis through a microRNA (miR-130a) that down-regulates antiangiogenic homeobox genes *GAX* and *HOXA5*. Blood 2008;111(3):1217–26.

[32] Anand S, Majeti BK, Acevedo LM, Murphy EA, Mukthavaram R, Scheppke L, Huang M, Shields DJ, Lindquist JN, Lapinski PE, King PD, Weis SM, Cheresh DA. MicroRNA-132-mediated loss of p120RasGAP activates the endothelium to facilitate pathological angiogenesis. Nat Med 2010;16(8):909–14.

[33] Liu A, Huang C, Cai X, Xu J, Yang D. Twist promotes angiogenesis in pancreatic cancer by targeting miR-497/VEGFA axis. Oncotarget 2016;7(18):25801–14.

[34] Cha ST, Chen PS, Johansson G, Chu CY, Wang MY, Jeng YM, Yu SL, Chen JS, Chang KJ, Jee SH, Tan CT, Lin MT, Kuo ML. MicroRNA-519c suppresses hypoxia-inducible factor-1α expression and tumor angiogenesis. Cancer Res 2010;70(7):2675–85.

[35] van Mil A, Grundmann S, Goumans MJ, Lei Z, Oerlemans MI, Jaksani S, Doevendans PA, Sluijter JP. MicroRNA-214 inhibits angiogenesis by targeting Quaking and reducing angiogenic growth factor release. Cardiovasc Res 2012;93(4):655–65.

[36] Chan YC, Khanna S, Roy S, Sen CK. miR-200b targets Ets-1 and is down-regulated by hypoxia to induce angiogenic response of endothelial cells. J Biol Chem 2011;286(3):2047–56.

[37] Pecot CV, Rupaimoole R, Yang D, Akbani R, Ivan C, Lu C, Wu S, Han HD, Shah MY, Rodriguez-Aguayo C, Bottsford-Miller J, Liu Y, Kim SB, Unruh A, Gonzalez-Villasana V, Huang L, Zand B, Moreno-Smith M, Mangala LS, Taylor M, Dalton HJ, Sehgal V, Wen Y, Kang Y, Baggerly

KA, Lee JS, Ram PT, Ravoori MK, Kundra V, Zhang X, Ali-Fehmi R, Gonzalez-Angulo AM, Massion PP, Calin GA, Lopez-Berestein G, Zhang W, Sood AK. Tumour angiogenesis regulation by the miR-200 family. Nat Commun 2013;4:2427.

[38] Chen L, Li ZY, Xu SY, Zhang XJ, Zhang Y, Luo K, Li WP. Upregulation of miR-107 inhibits glioma angiogenesis and VEGF expression. Cell Mol Neurobiol 2016;36(1):113–20.

[39] Sun CY, She XM, Qin Y, Chu ZB, Chen L, Ai LS, Zhang L, Hu Y. miR-15a and miR-16 affect the angiogenesis of multiple myeloma by targeting VEGF. Carcinogenesis 2013;34(2):426–35.

[40] Chamorro-Jorganes A, Araldi E, Penalva LO, Sandhu D, Fernandez-Hernando C, Suarez Y. MicroRNA-16 and microRNA-424 regulate cell-autonomous angiogenic functions in endothelial cells via targeting vascular endothelial growth factor receptor-2 and fibroblast growth factor receptor-1. Arterioscler Thromb Vasc Biol 2011;31(11):2595–606.

[41] He J, Jing Y, Li W, Qian X, Xu Q, Li FS, Liu LZ, Jiang BH, Jiang Y. Roles and mechanism of miR-199a and miR-125b in tumor angiogenesis. PLoS One 2013;8(2):e56647.

[42] Kanitz A, Imig J, Dziunycz PJ, Primorac A, Galgano A, Hofbauer GF, Gerber AP, Detmar M. The expression levels of microRNA-361-5p and its target VEGFA are inversely correlated in human cutaneous squamous cell carcinoma. PLoS One 2012;7(11):e49568.

[43] Stahlhut C, Suarez Y, Lu J, Mishima Y, Giraldez AJ. miR-1 and miR-206 regulate angiogenesis by modulating VegfA expression in zebrafish. Development 2012;139(23):4356–64.

[44] Zhou B, Ma R, Si W, Li S, Xu Y, Tu X, Wang Q. MicroRNA-503 targets FGF2 and VEGFA and inhibits tumor angiogenesis and growth. Cancer Lett 2013;333(2):159–69.

[45] Yang X, Zhang XF, Lu X, Jia HL, Liang L, Dong QZ, Ye QH, Qin LX. MicroRNA-26a suppresses angiogenesis in human hepatocellular carcinoma by targeting hepatocyte growth factor-cMet pathway. Hepatology 2014;59(5):1874–85.

[46] Bernardo BC, Gao XM, Winbanks CE, Boey EJ, Tham YK, Kiriazis H, Gregorevic P, Obad S, Kauppinen S, Du XJ, Lin RC, McMullen JR. Therapeutic inhibition of the miR-34 family attenuates pathological cardiac remodeling and improves heart function. Proc Natl Acad Sci USA 2012;109(43):17615–20.

[47] Wang Y, Sun B, Sun H, Zhao X, Wang X, Zhao N, Zhang Y, Li Y, Gu Q, Liu F, Shao B, An J. Regulation of proliferation, angiogenesis and apoptosis in hepatocellular carcinoma by miR-26b-5p. Tumour Biol 2016;37(8):10965–79.

[48] Han S, Kong YC, Sun B, Han QH, Chen Y, Wang YC. microRNA-218 inhibits oxygen-induced retinal neovascularization via reducing the expression of roundabout 1. Chin Med J (Engl) 2016;129(6):709–15.

[49] Shen H, Wang L, Ge X, Jiang CF, Shi ZM, Li DM, Liu WT, Yu X, Shu YQ. MicroRNA-137 inhibits tumor growth and sensitizes chemosensitivity to paclitaxel and cisplatin in lung cancer. Oncotarget 2016;7(15):20728–42.

[50] Gao F, Sun M, Gong Y, Wang H, Wang Y, Hou H. MicroRNA-195a-3p inhibits angiogenesis by targeting MMP2 in murine mesenchymal stem cells. Mol Reprod Dev 2016;83(5):413–23.

[51] Ma H, Pan JS, Jin LX, Wu J, Ren YD, Chen P, Xiao C, Han J. MicroRNA-17~92 inhibits colorectal cancer progression by targeting angiogenesis. Cancer Lett 2016;376(2):293–302.

[52] Jiang CF, Li DM, Shi ZM, Wang L, Liu MM, Ge X, Liu X, Qian YC, Wen YY, Zhen LL, Lin J, Liu LZ, Jiang BH. Estrogen regulates miRNA expression: implication of estrogen receptor and miR-124/AKT2 in tumor growth and angiogenesis. Oncotarget 2016;7(24):36940-55.

[53] Poliseno L, Tuccoli A, Mariani L, Evangelista M, Citti L, Woods K, Mercatanti A, Hammond S, Rainaldi G. MicroRNAs modulate the angiogenic properties of HUVECs. Blood 2006;108(9):3068–71.

[54] le Sage C, Nagel R, Egan DA, Schrier M, Mesman E, Mangiola A, Anile C, Maira G, Mercatelli N, Ciafre SA, Farace MG, Agami R. Regulation of the p27[Kip1] tumor suppressor by miR-221 and miR-222 promotes cancer cell proliferation. EMBO J 2007;26(15):3699–708.

[55] Suarez Y, Fernandez-Hernando C, Pober JS, Sessa WC. Dicer dependent microRNAs regulate gene expression and functions in human endothelial cells. Circ Res 2007;100(8):1164–73.

[56] Ghosh G, Subramanian IV, Adhikari N, Zhang X, Joshi HP, Basi D, Chandrashekhar YS, Hall JL, Roy S, Zeng Y, Ramakrishnan S. Hypoxia-induced microRNA-424 expression in human endothelial cells regulates HIF-α isoforms and promotes angiogenesis. J Clin Invest 2010;120(11):4141–54.

[57] Hu J, Ni S, Cao Y, Zhang T, Wu T, Yin X, Lang Y, Lu H. The angiogenic effect of microRNA-21 targeting TIMP3 through the regulation of MMP2 and MMP9. PLoS One 2016;11(2):e0149537.

[58] Hermansen SK, Nielsen BS, Aaberg-Jessen C, Kristensen BW. miR-21 is linked to glioma angiogenesis: a co-localization study. J Histochem Cytochem 2016;64(2):138–48.

[59] Liu LZ, Li C, Chen Q, Jing Y, Carpenter R, Jiang Y, Kung HF, Lai L, Jiang BH. MiR-21 induced angiogenesis through AKT and ERK activation and HIF-1α expression. PLoS One 2011;6(4):e19139.

[60] Polytarchou C, Iliopoulos D, Hatziapostolou M, Kottakis F, Maroulakou I, Struhl K, Tsichlis PN. Akt2 regulates all Akt isoforms and promotes resistance to hypoxia through induction of miR-21 upon oxygen deprivation. Cancer Res 2011;71(13):4720–31.

[61] Isanejad A, Alizadeh AM, Amani Shalamzari S, Khodayari H, Khodayari S, Khori V, Khojastehnjad N. MicroRNA-206, let-7a and microRNA-21 pathways involved in the anti-angiogenesis effects of the interval exercise training and hormone therapy in breast cancer. Life Sci 2016;151:30–40.

[62] Svobodova E, Kubikova J, Svoboda P. Production of small RNAs by mammalian Dicer. Pflugers Arch 2016;468:1089–102.

[63] Yang WJ, Yang DD, Na S, Sandusky GE, Zhang Q, Zhao G. Dicer is required for embryonic angiogenesis during mouse development. J Biol Chem 2005;280(10):9330–5.

[64] Zhang J, Li S, Li L, Li M, Guo C, Yao J, Mi S. Exosome and exosomal microRNA: trafficking, sorting, and function. Genomics Proteomics Bioinformatics 2015;13(1):17–24.

[65] Giraldez AJ, Cinalli RM, Glasner ME, Enright AJ, Thomson JM, Baskerville S, Hammond SM, Bartel DP, Schier AF. MicroRNAs regulate brain morphogenesis in zebrafish. Science 2005;308(5723):833–8.

[66] Suarez Y, Fernandez-Hernando C, Yu J, Gerber SA, Harrison KD, Pober JS, Iruela-Arispe ML, Merkenschlager M, Sessa WC. Dicer-dependent endothelial microRNAs are necessary for postnatal angiogenesis. Proc Natl Acad Sci USA 2008;105(37):14082–7.

[67] Nicoli S, Standley C, Walker P, Hurlstone A, Fogarty KE, Lawson ND. MicroRNA-mediated integration of haemodynamics and Vegf signalling during angiogenesis. Nature 2010;464(7292):1196–200.

[68] Png KJ, Halberg N, Yoshida M, Tavazoie SF. A microRNA regulon that mediates endothelial recruitment and metastasis by cancer cells. Nature 2012;481(7380):190–4.

[69] Katare R, Riu F, Mitchell K, Gubernator M, Campagnolo P, Cui Y, Fortunato O, Avolio E, Cesselli D, Beltrami AP, Angelini G, Emanueli C, Madeddu P. Transplantation of human pericyte progenitor cells improves the repair of infarcted heart through activation of an angiogenic program involving micro-RNA-132. Circ Res 2011;109(8):894–906.

[70] Lagos D, Pollara G, Henderson S, Gratrix F, Fabani M, Milne RS, Gotch F, Boshoff C. miR-132 regulates antiviral innate immunity through suppression of the p300 transcriptional co-activator. Nat Cell Biol 2010;12(5):513–9.

[71] Mulik S, Xu J, Reddy PB, Rajasagi NK, Gimenez F, Sharma S, Lu PY, Rouse BT. Role of miR-132 in angiogenesis after ocular infection with herpes simplex virus. Am J Pathol 2012;181(2):525–34.

[72] Ge XT, Lei P, Wang HC, Zhang AL, Han ZL, Chen X, Li SH, Jiang RC, Kang CS, Zhang JN. miR-21 improves the neurological outcome after traumatic brain injury in rats. Sci Rep 2014;4:6718.

[73] Tomanek RJ, Busch TL. Coordinated capillary and myocardial growth in response to thyroxine treatment. Anat Rec 1998;251(1):44–9.

[74] Bergh JJ, Lin HY, Lansing L, Mohamed SN, Davis FB, Mousa S, Davis PJ. Integrin $\alpha v \beta 3$ contains a cell surface receptor site for thyroid hormone that is linked to activation of mitogen-activated protein kinase and induction of angiogenesis. Endocrinology 2005;146(7):2864–71.

[75] Luidens MK, Mousa SA, Davis FB, Lin HY, Davis PJ. Thyroid hormone and angiogenesis. Vasc Pharmacol 2010;52(3–4):142–5.

[76] Davis PJ, Davis FB, Mousa SA, Luidens MK, Lin HY. Membrane receptor for thyroid hormone: physiologic and pharmacologic implications. Annu Rev Pharmacol Toxicol 2011;51:99–115.

[77] Davis FB, Mousa SA, O'Connor L, Mohamed S, Lin HY, Cao HJ, Davis PJ. Proangiogenic action of thyroid hormone is fibroblast growth factor-dependent and is initiated at the cell surface. Circ Res 2004;94(11):1500–6.

[78] Mousa SA, Lin HY, Tang HY, Hercbergs A, Luidens MK, Davis PJ. Modulation of angiogenesis by thyroid hormone and hormone analogues: implications for cancer management. Angiogenesis 2014;17(3):463–9.

[79] Cohen K, Flint N, Shalev S, Erez D, Baharal T, Davis PJ, Hercbergs A, Ellis M, Ashur-Fabian O. Thyroid hormone regulates adhesion, migration and matrix metalloproteinase 9 activity via $\alpha v \beta 3$ integrin in myeloma cells. Oncotarget 2014;5(15):6312–22.

[80] Mousa SA, Thangirala S, Lin HY, Tang HY, Glinsky GV, Davis PJ. MicroRNA-21 and microRNA-15A expression in human breast cancer (MDA-MB-231) cells exposed to nanoparticulate tetraiodothyroacetic acid (Nanotetrac). ENDO Annual Meeting; June 21–24, 2014; Chicago.

[81] Melnik BC. MiR-21: an environmental driver of malignant melanoma? J Transl Med 2015;13:202.

[82] Enquobahrie DA, Williams MA, Qiu C, Siscovick DS, Sorensen TK. Global maternal early pregnancy peripheral blood mRNA and miRNA expression profiles according to plasma 25-hydroxyvitamin D concentrations. J Matern Fetal Neonatal Med 2011;24(8):1002–12.

[83] Elmen J, Lindow M, Schutz S, Lawrence M, Petri A, Obad S, Lindholm M, Hedtjarn M, Hansen HF, Berger U, Gullans S, Kearney P, Sarnow P, Straarup EM, Kauppinen S. LNA-mediated microRNA silencing in non-human primates. Nature 2008;452(7189):896–9.

[84] Krutzfeldt J, Rajewsky N, Braich R, Rajeev KG, Tuschl T, Manoharan M, Stoffel M. Silencing of microRNAs in vivo with 'antagomirs'. Nature 2005;438(7068):685–9.

[85] Esau C, Davis S, Murray SF, Yu XX, Pandey SK, Pear M, Watts L, Booten SL, Graham M, McKay R, Subramaniam A, Propp S, Lollo BA, Freier S, Bennett CF, Bhanot S, Monia BP. miR-122 regulation of lipid metabolism revealed by in vivo antisense targeting. Cell Metab 2006;3(2):87–98.

[86] Ebert MS, Sharp PA. Emerging roles for natural microRNA sponges. Curr Biol 2010;20(19):R858–61.

[87] Bader AG. miR-34—a microRNA replacement therapy is headed to the clinic. Front Genet 2012;3:120.

[88] Ji J, Shi J, Budhu A, Yu Z, Forgues M, Roessler S, Ambs S, Chen Y, Meltzer PS, Croce CM, Qin LX, Man K, Lo CM, Lee J, Ng IO, Fan J, Tang ZY, Sun HC, Wang XW. MicroRNA expression, survival, and response to interferon in liver cancer. N Engl J Med 2009;361(15):1437–47.

CHAPTER 6

Naturally Occurring Angiogenesis Inhibitors

Shaker A. Mousa, Maii Abu Taleb and Paul J. Davis

Contents

INTRODUCTION

Angiogenesis is the product of dividing or sprouting of existing capillaries. Integrated proliferation, migration, adhesion, differentiation, and assembly of vascular endothelial cells and attendant vascular smooth muscle cells are essential to this process. These components of angiogenesis reflect interplay of proangiogenic factors—vascular endothelial growth factor (VEGF), fibroblast growth factor (FGF), platelet-derived growth factor (PDGF)—and anti-angiogenic factors. Angiogenesis is essential for wound healing and to repair the myocardium after ischemic damage. Disordered angiogenesis contributes to growth of solid tumors, hypertension, arthritis, diabetic retinopathy and, it is thought, to atherosclerosis.

The contribution of angiogenesis to atherosclerosis is controversial, but an association between intimal neovascularization and atherosclerosis was first reported in 1876 [1], and atherosclerotic plaque instability and rupture are consequences of the development of new vasa vasora [1–3]. The possibility of proangiogenic pharmacologic intercession in blood vessel disease of the heart and limbs was anticipated [4], but clinical trials of such intercessions

Anti-Angiogenesis Strategies in Cancer Therapies
http://dx.doi.org/10.1016/B978-0-12-802576-5.00006-1

have been inconclusive; further, vascular growth factors may carry a risk of destabilizing coronary artery plaques [5,6]. In contrast, the contribution of angiogenesis to solid tumor growth is not controversial, and anti-angiogenic therapeutic interventions in the setting of cancer have had some success.

NUTRACEUTICAL-DERIVED POLYPHENOL ANGIOGENESIS INHIBITORS

Plant phenols, for example, the flavonoids [7], are an important category of phytochemicals, and a number of these substances have been shown to have anti-angiogenic properties that are relevant to cancer. Among these are green tea polyphenols [epigallocatechin gallate (EGCG)] and soy bean isoflavones (genistein).

Curcumin, a plant-derived natural polyphenol, has some promise as an anti-cancer drug and shows synergistic effects with cytotoxic agents. Studies on gemcitabine-resistant patients with pancreatic cancer who received 8 g oral curcumin daily in combination with gemcitabine-based chemotherapy showed that the combination was safe and that additional evaluation of its efficacy is needed [8]. Transcription of the genes for epidermal growth factor receptor (EGFR), VEGFR-1, VEGFR-2, and VEGFR-3 and for matrix metalloproteinases MMP-2 and MMP-9 is downregulated by curcumin. Curcumin also inhibits Src and focal adhesion kinase (FAK) activities relevant to induction of proangiogenic genes. Finally, this phenol also inhibits endothelial cell migration. These actions combine to suppress proliferation and invasiveness of tumor cells in culture and in xenografts [9].

The pharmacological action of tea is mainly attributed to large quantities of polyphenolic compounds known as catechins, which include epicatechin (EC), epigallocatechin (EGC), epicatechin-3 gallate (ECG), and EGCG, particularly in green tea. Tea polyphenols suppress proliferation of capillary endothelial cells, apparently via several signal transduction pathways, and in human breast cancer cells EGCG treatment reduced MMP-2 activity, as well as the expression of FAK, membrane type 1-MMP, nuclear factor kappa B (NFκB), VEGF, and the adhesion of cells to the extra-cellular matrix (ECM) [9]. These polyphenols have been shown to reduce growth of prostate cancer xenografts. Administration of green tea polyphenols orally to transgenic mice with adenocarcinoma of the prostate (TRAMP mice) for 32 weeks has been shown to markedly reduce prostate cancer growth and distant site metastases [10]. The green tea effect is associated with a decrease in cell proliferation and an increase in apoptosis in prostate tissue, a favorable change in the insulin-like growth factor (IGF) axis, and significant suppression of angiogenic and metastatic markers [7]. Green tea as prostate cancer chemoprevention was associated with changes in systemic biomarkers that indicated some efficacy of this approach [7]. Such activity appeared to be independent of bioaccumulation. Fig. 6.1 summarizes naturally occurring anti-angiogenesis substances.

Loading of poly(lactide-co-glycolide) (PLGA) nanoparticles with the green tea polyphenol EGCG results in a 10-fold dose advantage over unmodified EGCG in terms of proapoptotic and anti-angiogenic effects [7] on which the chemo-preventive effects of EGCG depend in both in vitro and in vivo systems [11].

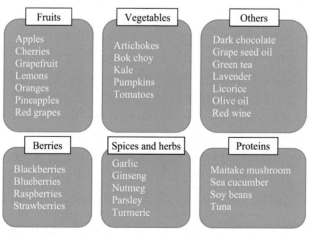

Figure 6.1 *Foods rich with naturally occurring anti-angiogenic substances.*

Fucosylated chondroitin sulfate (FCS) is a heparin-like gly-cosaminoglycan (GAG) isolated form sea cucumbers. Recent studies have demonstrated that FCS possesses various biological activities, such as anti-coagulant, anti-thrombotic, and anti-viral effects. Importantly, FCS showed remarkable function as an inhibitor of metastasis and thrombosis in mouse melanoma activity by the NFκB/tissue factor/factor Xa pathway [12]. Additionally, FCS was able to suppress metastasis and inflammatory reaction by blocking of selectin activity. Low-molecular-weight fucosylated chondroitin sulfate (LFCS) prepared from the native FCS was demonstrated to inhibit Lewis lung carcinoma growth and metastasis in a dose-dependent manner in vivo. The anti-cancer activity was related to p53/p21-induced cell cycle arrest, caspase-3-induced apoptosis, VEGF-mediated angiogenesis, and TIMP/MMPs-mediated metastasis via the ERK1/2/p38MAPK/NFκB pathway [13].

Resveratrol, a dietary polyphenol derived from grapes, berries, peanuts, and other plant sources, has been shown to affect several steps in the tumorigenic process, including tumor-related angiogenesis [9]. Resveratrol inhibits capillary endothelial cell growth and new blood vessel growth in animals. It also prevents diethyl nitrosamine-initiated and phenobarbital-promoted hepatic carcinogenesis in rats by interrupting cell proliferation, inducing apoptosis and impeding angiogenesis. The latter is achieved by suppressing VEGF expression through downregulation of hypoxia induced factor-1α (HIF-1α) gene expression. Furthermore, the synthetic stilbene derivatives of resveratrol have a stronger inhibitory effect on angiogenesis than unmodified resveratrol, as measured with cell proliferation and tube formation in bovine aorta endothelial cells [14].

Inhibition of tumorigenesis by flavonoids depends on anti-angiogenesis, anti-tumor cell proliferation, and anti-oxidant effects. Stromal cells may also be affected by flavonoids. These polyphenols inhibit reactive oxygen species (ROS) generation and hypoxia-signaling cascades. They also decrease cyclooxygenase (COX-2) activity and disrupt EGFR, insulin-like growth factor receptor-1 (IGFR-1), and NFκB signaling pathways [15] that are relevant to angiogenesis.

MARINE NONGLYCOSAMINOGLYCAN SULFATED GLYCANS

Glycosaminoglycans (GAGs) are carbohydrates that have desirable therapeutic effects on pathologic thrombosis, neovascularization, cancer, and inflammation. The most commonly used GAGs in clinical practice are heparin, chondroitin sulfate, and keratin sulfate, but these compounds have significant disadvantages [16].

Non-GAG sulfated glycans now are also available. Examples of these are marine sulfated fucans (SFs) and sulfated galactans (SGs). The chemical structures of these glycans are oligosaccharide repeating units and distinct from those of GAGs; SFs and SGs also have certain effects that differ from those of GAGs [17]. The SFs or SGs harvested from invertebrates and red algae are, compared to GAGs, homogeneous in terms of monosaccharide backbone constitution and patterns of sulfation.

Effects of the marine sulfated glycans that may be shown to be clinically advantageous are their development as anti-coagulant alternatives to heparin, particularly in those settings in which heparin is suboptimally effective or inactive. These sulfated glycans are a basis for defining the structure-activity relationships (SARs) of the family. Table 6.1 summarizes the activities of naturally occurring GAGs with anti-angiogenesis and anti-inflammatory activities.

NATURAL LIPID PRODUCTS

Arachidonic acid (AA) is a homeostatically important omega-6 long-chain, polyunsaturated fatty acid that in humans is primarily derived from diet [18,19]. Certain lipid mediators, such as epoxyeicosatrienoic acids (EETs), have recently been recognized to be

Table 6.1 Biological effects of natural glycosaminoglycan from animals and marine sources

Anti-angiogenesis and anti-cancer	- Inhibition activities on growth factors necessary for cell differentiation and neovascularization - Inhibition activities on selectins necessary for cell migration, attachment, and adhesion
Anti-inflammation	- Inhibition of l-selectin during leukocyte recruitment and rolling - Inhibition of chemokine functions in leukocyte activation - Decreased extravasation of activated leukocytes - Inhibition of binding of free chemokines to infiltrated leukocytes in inflamed tissues - Completion with hydrolase activity during ECM processing necessary to enhance leukocyte transmigration. Marine sulfated glycans may be less active or inactive in this context.

Some natural glycosaminoglycans possess anti-coagulant activities and others are devoid of such activities.
Source: Modified from Table 3 of Pomin VH. Marine non-glycosaminoglycan sulfated glycans as potential pharmaceuticals. Pharmaceuticals 2015;8(4):848–64. Used under the terms and conditions of the Creative Commons Attribution license.

derived from AA. They are produced by the liver via the cytochrome P450 enzyme pathway. EETs have anti-angiogenic, anti-inflammatory, and anti-atherosclerotic properties [20,21]. Aside from these desirable qualities, EETs may detrimentally support myocardial fibrosis [22]. Other derivatives of AA include lysophosphatidylcholine (LPC) and lysophosphatic acid (LPA) [23] and lipoxins and 15 deoxy-prostaglandin D2. The latter is the ligand of peroxisome proliferator-activated receptor (PPAR)-γ. Anti-inflammatory qualities are exhibited by these lipid mediators [18]. Several AA-derived lipid mediators with known proangiogenesis properties have been examined in order to define how interactions of lipid metabolites with one another and metabolism of lipids affect angiogenesis that is relevant to cancer and cardiovascular events [19].

Actions of AA-derived metabolites/lipid mediators [24–26] on angiogenesis have been studied in the in vivo chick chorioallantoic membrane (CAM) model system [27]. LPA, LPC, and the EETs were found to be proangiogenic, while 15 deoxy-PGJ2 and 15 epi-lipoxin A4 inhibited angiogenesis promoted by AA-derived and non-AA derived lipid mediators. The mediators examined have specific mechanisms of action that influence pathways that intersect with atherosclerotic and angiogenic processes [28–31].

Among the EETs tested, the 5,6-; 8,9-; 11,12-; and 14,15-structures have been shown to be proangiogenic. They stimulate endothelial cell migration and the generation of capillary-like structures [24–26]. Enzymatic hydration is required to achieve the proangiogenic activities of 5,6- and 8,9-EET. Interestingly, increased intracellular concentrations of EETs result in endothelial cells when VEGF stimulates angiogenesis through increasing CYP2C promoter activity [32]. An EET antagonist, 14,15-epoxyeicosa-5(Z)-enoic acid (14,15-EEZE), blocks endothelial cell tube formation induced by VEGF. Enhancement of VEGF-stimulated endothelial cell sprouting can be opposed by CYP2C anti-sense nucleotides. Such results indicated that EETs derived from CYP2C function as second messengers and that decreased VEGF responsiveness results when increases in CYP activity are blocked. Over-expression of CYP2C9 has been shown to stimulate endothelial tube formation, and induction by CYP2C9 of 11,12-EET may increase COX-2 expression [33].

Bioactive lysophospholipids LPA and sphingosine-1-phosphate (S1P) are generated from phospholipid precursors of membranes and are elaborated by platelets [34–36], macrophages [34,37], and certain types of cancer cells [34,38]. Endothelial cell migration and proliferation are regulated by LPA and S1P [34,39], acting through G protein-coupled receptors linked to the endothelial differentiation gene (Edg) family [40,41] and intracellular signaling factors, such as inositol phosphates and intracellular calcium [42], adenylyl cyclase [43], protein kinase C (PKC), and other signaling pathways [34,44,45]. Different LPC and LPA acyl moieties may have different effects on target cells [46]. That is, unsaturated LPA species (16:1 LPA, 18:1, an unsaturated LPA found in high concentration in human serum, and 18:2 LPA) cause dedifferentiation of vascular smooth muscle cells, but saturated LPA species do not [46,47].

The 15 epi-lipoxin A4 analog, 15 epi-16 (paraflouro)-(phenoxy-lipoxin A(4) (ATL-1), inhibits angiogenesis in the cultured human umbilical vein endothelial cell (HUVEC) model. This is a result of reductions in VEGF-stimulated cell proliferation, in MMP-9 activity, and impaired generation of the actin cytoskeleton [48]. ATL-1 has been reported to reduce inflammation-linked angiogenesis by 50% [49]. It blocks endothelial cell adhesion to fibronectin. In addition, aspirin-triggered 15 epi-lipoxin A4 and its native enantiomer, lipoxin A4, are very anti-inflammatory by mechanisms that are receptor-, cell-type-, and tissue-specific [48]. The functional mechanisms by which 15 epi-lipoxin A4 act include reductions in neutrophil chemotaxis and reduction in neutrophil diapedesis from postcapillary venules. Relevant to angiogenesis, 15 epi-lipoxin A4 and lipoxin A4 analogs inhibit release of certain cytokines and chemokines [50]. The molecular mechanisms involved in these actions of lipoxin A4 analogs' effects at the level of transcription have been explored [51], as well as their actions on inhibition of VEGF-stimulated production of interleukin (IL)-6, of tumor necrosis factor (TNF)-α, interferon (IFN)-γ, IL-8, and of inter-cellular adhesion molecule (ICAM)-1 expression [52].

The anti-angiogenic activity of 15-deoxy-PGJ2 involves activation of PPAR-γ by 15-deoxy-PGJ2, and consequent suppression of HUVEC differentiation has been described [53]. PPAR-γ activation also inhibits the proliferative effects of exogenous vascular growth factors in in vitro models and downregulates angiogenesis in vivo in a rat cornea model [30]. Reduced levels of mRNAs of vascular endothelial cell growth factor receptors 1 (Flt-1) and 2 (Flk/KDR) and urokinase plasminogen activator also result from treatment of HUVECs with 15 deoxy-PGJ2. A 15 deoxy-PGJ2 effect to increase plasminogen activator inhibitor-1 (PAI-1) mRNA abundance may also explain its anti-angiogenesis activity [30]. In addition, pretreatment of endothelial cells with lipoxin A4 reduces VEGF-stimulated VEGF receptor 2 (KDR/FLK-1) phosphorylation and specific signaling events, including activation of ERK1/2, and Akt [52].

AA-derived angiogenesis inhibitors, such as 15 epi-lipoxin A4 or 15 deoxy-PGJ2 exhibit a broad spectrum of anti-angiogenesis effects against multiple, various proangiogenesis factors. This is in contrast to single mechanism-based interventions, such as anti-VEGF. Thus, AA-derived products have attractiveness as angiogenesis-modifying interventions.

In summary, in vivo angiogenesis models document that extensive interplay exists between potent lipid mediators originating from polyunsaturated, omega-6 AA. These mediators are derived from metabolic pathways that interface with actions of a variety of medications, with genetics, and with other factors that are involved in pathogenesis of human diseases. Much additional research is warranted on lipid regulators that have anti- and proangiogenic properties.

REFERENCES

[1] Khurana R, Simons M, Martin JF, Zachary IC. Role of angiogenesis in cardiovascular disease: a critical appraisal. Circulation 2005;112(12): 1813–24.

[2] O'Brien ER, Garvin MR, Dev R, Stewart DK, Hinohara T, Simpson JB, Schwartz SM. Angiogenesis in human coronary atherosclerotic plaques. Am J Pathol 1994;145(4):883–94.

[3] Sueishi K, Yonemitsu Y, Nakagawa K, Kaneda Y, Kumamoto M, Nakashima Y. Atherosclerosis and angiogenesis. Its pathophysiological significance in humans as well as in an animal model induced by the gene transfer of vascular endothelial growth factor. Ann NY Acad Sci 1997;811:311–22. 22-24.

[4] Simons M, Ware JA. Therapeutic angiogenesis in cardiovascular disease. Nat Rev Drug Discov 2003;2(11):863–71.

[5] Celletti FL, Waugh JM, Amabile PG, Brendolan A, Hilfiker PR, Dake MD. Vascular endothelial growth factor enhances atherosclerotic plaque progression. Nat Med 2001;7(4):425–9.

[6] Moulton KS, Heller E, Konerding MA, Flynn E, Palinski W, Folkman J. Angiogenesis inhibitors endostatin or TNP-470 reduce intimal neovascularization and plaque growth in apolipoprotein E-deficient mice. Circulation 1999;99(13):1726–32.

[7] Siddiqui IA, Adhami VM, Bharali DJ, Hafeez BB, Asim M, Khwaja SI, Ahmad N, Cui H, Mousa SA, Mukhtar H. Introducing nanochemoprevention as a novel approach for cancer control: proof of principle with green tea polyphenol epigallocatechin-3-gallate. Cancer Res 2009;69(5):1712–6.

[8] Kanai M, Yoshimura K, Asada M, Imaizumi A, Suzuki C, Matsumoto S, Nishimura T, Mori Y, Masui T, Kawaguchi Y, Yanagihara K, Yazumi S, Chiba T, Guha S, Aggarwal BB. A phase I/II study of gemcitabine-based chemotherapy plus curcumin for patients with gemcitabine-resistant pancreatic cancer. Cancer Chemoth Pharm 2011;68(1):157–64.

[9] Wang Z, Dabrosin C, Yin X, Fuster MM, Arreola A, Rathmell WK, Generali D, Nagaraju GP, El-Rayes B, Ribatti D, Chen YC, Honoki K, Fujii H, Georgakilas AG, Nowsheen S, Amedei A, Niccolai E, Amin A, Ashraf SS, Helferich B, Yang X, Guha G, Bhakta D, Ciriolo MR, Aquilano K, Chen S, Halicka D, Mohammed SI, Azmi AS, Bilsland A, Keith WN, Jensen LD. Broad targeting of angiogenesis for cancer prevention and therapy. Semin Cancer Biol 2015;35(Suppl.):S224–43.

[10] Gupta S, Hastak K, Ahmad N, Lewin JS, Mukhtar H. Inhibition of prostate carcinogenesis in TRAMP mice by oral infusion of green tea polyphenols. Proc Natl Acad Sci USA 2001;98(18):10350–5.

[11] Nguyen MM, Ahmann FR, Nagle RB, Hsu CH, Tangrea JA, Parnes HL, Sokoloff MH, Gretzer MB, Chow HH. Randomized, double-blind, placebo-controlled trial of polyphenon E in prostate cancer patients before prostatectomy: evaluation of potential chemopreventive activities. Cancer Prev Res (Phila) 2012;5(2):290–8.

[12] Zhao Y, Zhang D, Wang S, Tao L, Wang A, Chen W, Zhu Z, Zheng S, Gao X, Lu Y. Holothurian glycosaminoglycan inhibits metastasis and thrombosis via targeting of nuclear factor-κB/tissue factor/Factor Xa pathway in melanoma B16F10 cells. PLoS One 2013;8(2):e56557.

[13] Liu X, Liu Y, Hao J, Zhao X, Lang Y, Fan F, Cai C, Li G, Zhang L, Yu G. In vivo anti-cancer mechanism of low-molecular-weight fucosylated chondroitin sulfate (LFCS) from sea cucumber cucumaria frondosa. Molecules 2016;21(5):1–12.

[14] Marti-Centelles R, Cejudo-Marin R, Falomir E, Murga J, Carda M, Marco JA. Inhibition of VEGF expression in cancer cells and endothelial cell differentiation by synthetic stilbene derivatives. Bioorg Med Chem 2013;21(11):3010–5.

[15] van Meeteren ME, Hendriks JJ, Dijkstra CD, van Tol EA. Dietary compounds prevent oxidative damage and nitric oxide production by cells involved in demyelinating disease. Biochem Pharmacol 2004;67(5):967–75.

[16] Pomin VH. Marine non-glycosaminoglycan sulfated glycans as potential pharmaceuticals. Pharmaceuticals 2015;8(4):848–64.

[17] Pomin VH. Fucanomics and galactanomics: current status in drug discovery, mechanisms of action and role of the well-defined structures. Biochim Biophys Acta 2012;1820(12):1971–9.

[18] Serhan CN, Chiang N, Van Dyke TE. Resolving inflammation: dual anti-inflammatory and pro-resolution lipid mediators. Nat Rev Immunol 2008;8(5):349–61.

[19] Hjelte LE, Nilsson A. Arachidonic acid and ischemic heart disease. J Nutr 2005;135(9):2271–3.

[20] Gauthier KM, Yang W, Gross GJ, Campbell WB. Roles of epoxyeicosatrienoic acids in vascular regulation and cardiac preconditioning. J Cardiovasc Pharmacol 2007;50(6):601–8.

[21] Wray J, Bishop-Bailey D. Epoxygenases and peroxisome proliferator-activated receptors in mammalian vascular biology. Exp Physiol 2008;93(1):148–54.

[22] Levick SP, Loch DC, Taylor SM, Janicki JS. Arachidonic acid metabolism as a potential mediator of cardiac fibrosis associated with inflammation. J Immunol 2007;178(2):641–6.

[23] Aoki J. Mechanisms of lysophosphatidic acid production. Semin Cell Dev Biol 2004;15(5):477–89.

[24] Fleming I. Epoxyeicosatrienoic acids, cell signaling and angiogenesis. Prostaglandins Other Lipid Mediat 2007;82(1-4):60–7.

[25] Spector AA. Arachidonic acid cytochrome P450 epoxygenase pathway. J Lipid Res 2009;50(Suppl.):S52–6.

[26] Pozzi A, Popescu V, Yang S, Mei S, Shi M, Puolitaival SM, Caprioli RM, Capdevila JH. The anti-tumorigenic properties of peroxisomal proliferator-activated receptor α are arachidonic acid epoxygenase-mediated. J Biol Chem 2010;285(17):12840–50.

[27] Glew RH, Okolie H, Huang YS, Chuang LT, Suberu O, Crossey M, VanderJagt DJ. Abnormalities in the fatty-acid composition of the serum phospholipids of stroke patients. J Natl Med Assoc 2004;96(6):826–32.

[28] Mills GB, Moolenaar WH. The emerging role of lysophosphatidic acid in cancer. Nat Rev Cancer 2003;3(8):582–91.

[29] Cezar-de-Mello PF, Vieira AM, Nascimento-Silva V, Villela CG, Barja-Fidalgo C, Fierro IM. ATL-1, an analogue of aspirin-triggered lipoxin A_4, is a potent inhibitor of several steps in angiogenesis induced by vascular endothelial growth factor. Br J Pharmacol 2008;153(5):956–65.

[30] Xin X, Yang S, Kowalski J, Gerritsen ME. Peroxisome proliferator-activated receptor gamma ligands are potent inhibitors of angiogenesis in vitro and in vivo. J Biol Chem 1999;274(13):9116–21.

[31] Pozzi A, Macias-Perez I, Abair T, Wei S, Su Y, Zent R, Falck JR, Capdevila JH. Characterization of 5,6- and 8,9-epoxyeicosatrienoic acids

(5,6- and 8,9-EET) as potent in vivo angiogenic lipids. J Biol Chem 2005;280(29):27138–46.

[32] Webler AC, Michaelis UR, Popp R, Barbosa-Sicard E, Murugan A, Falck JR, Fisslthaler B, Fleming I. Epoxyeicosatrienoic acids are part of the VEGF-activated signaling cascade leading to angiogenesis. Am J Physiol Cell Physiol 2008;295(5):C1292–301.

[33] Michaelis UR, Falck JR, Schmidt R, Busse R, Fleming I. Cytochrome P4502C9-derived epoxyeicosatrienoic acids induce the expression of cyclooxygenase-2 in endothelial cells. Arterioscler Thromb Vasc Biol 2005;25(2):321–6.

[34] Wu WT, Chen CN, Lin CI, Chen JH, Lee H. Lysophospholipids enhance matrix metalloproteinase-2 expression in human endothelial cells. Endocrinology 2005;146(8):3387–400.

[35] Gerrard JM, Robinson P. Identification of the molecular species of lysophosphatidic acid produced when platelets are stimulated by thrombin. Biochim Biophys Acta 1989;1001(3):282–5.

[36] Gaits F, Fourcade O, Le Balle F, Gueguen G, Gaige B, Gassama-Diagne A, Fauvel J, Salles JP, Mauco G, Simon MF, Chap H. Lysophosphatidic acid as a phospholipid mediator: pathways of synthesis. FEBS Lett 1997;410(1):54–8.

[37] Lee H, Liao JJ, Graeler M, Huang MC, Goetzl EJ. Lysophospholipid regulation of mononuclear phagocytes. Biochim Biophys Acta 2002;1582(1-3):175–7.

[38] Shen Z, Belinson J, Morton RE, Xu Y. Phorbol 12-myristate 13-acetate stimulates lysophosphatidic acid secretion from ovarian and cervical cancer cells but not from breast or leukemia cells. Gynecol Oncol 1998;71(3):364–8.

[39] Spiegel S, Merrill AH Jr. Sphingolipid metabolism and cell growth regulation. FASEB J 1996;10(12):1388–97.

[40] Panchatcharam M, Miriyala S, Yang F, Rojas M, End C, Vallant C, Dong A, Lynch K, Chun J, Morris AJ, Smyth SS. Lysophosphatidic acid receptors 1 and 2 play roles in regulation of vascular injury responses but not blood pressure. Circ Res 2008;103(6):662–70.

[41] Moolenaar WH. Bioactive lysophospholipids and their G protein-coupled receptors. Exp Cell Res 1999;253(1):230–8.

[42] An S, Bleu T, Zheng Y, Goetzl EJ. Recombinant human G protein-coupled lysophosphatidic acid receptors mediate intracellular calcium mobilization. Mol Pharmacol 1998;54(5):881–8.

[43] Tigyi G, Fischer DJ, Sebok A, Marshall F, Dyer DL, Miledi R. Lysophosphatidic acid-induced neurite retraction in PC12 cells: neurite-protective effects of cyclic AMP signaling. J Neurochem 1996;66(2):549–58.

[44] Stahle M, Veit C, Bachfischer U, Schierling K, Skripczynski B, Hall A, Gierschik P, Giehl K. Mechanisms in LPA-induced tumor cell migration: critical role of phosphorylated ERK. J Cell Sci 2003;116(Pt 18):3835–46.

[45] Seewald S, Schmitz U, Seul C, Ko Y, Sachinidis A, Vetter H. Lysophosphatidic acid stimulates protein kinase C isoforms α, β, ϵ, and ζ in a pertussis toxin sensitive pathway in vascular smooth muscle cells. Am J Hypertens 1999;12(5):532–7.

[46] Hayashi K, Takahashi M, Nishida W, Yoshida K, Ohkawa Y, Kitabatake A, Aoki J, Arai H, Sobue K. Phenotypic modulation of vascular smooth muscle cells induced by unsaturated lysophosphatidic acids. Circ Res 2001;89(3):251–8.

[47] Yoshida K, Nishida W, Hayashi K, Ohkawa Y, Ogawa A, Aoki J, Arai H, Sobue K. Vascular remodeling induced by naturally occurring unsaturated lysophosphatidic acid in vivo. Circulation 2003;108(14):1746–52.

[48] Cezar-de-Mello PF, Nascimento-Silva V, Villela CG, Fierro IM. Aspirin-triggered lipoxin A$_4$ inhibition of VEGF-induced endothelial cell migration involves actin polymerization and focal adhesion assembly. Oncogene 2006;25(1):122–9.

[49] Fierro IM, Kutok JL, Serhan CN. Novel lipid mediator regulators of endothelial cell proliferation and migration: aspirin-triggered-15R-lipoxin A$_4$ and lipoxin A$_4$. J Pharmacol Exp Ther 2002;300(2):385–92.

[50] Pouliot M, Serhan CN. Lipoxin A$_4$ and aspirin-triggered 15-epi-LXA$_4$ inhibit tumor necrosis factor-α-initiated neutrophil responses and trafficking: novel regulators of a cytokine-chemokine axis relevant to periodontal diseases. J Periodontal Res 1999;34(7):370–3.

[51] Gewirtz AT, McCormick B, Neish AS, Petasis NA, Gronert K, Serhan CN, Madara JL. Pathogen-induced chemokine secretion from model intestinal epithelium is inhibited by lipoxin A4 analogs. J Clin Invest 1998;101(9):1860–9.

[52] Baker N, O'Meara SJ, Scannell M, Maderna P, Godson C. Lipoxin A$_4$: anti-inflammatory and anti-angiogenic impact on endothelial cells. J Immunol 2009;182(6):3819–26.

[53] Imaizumi T, Matsumiya T, Tamo W, Shibata T, Fujimoto K, Kumagai M, Yoshida H, Cui XF, Tanji K, Hatakeyama M, Wakabayashi K, Satoh K. 15-Deoxy-D12,14-prostaglandin J2 inhibits CX3CL1/fractalkine expression in human endothelial cells. Immunol Cell Biol 2002;80(6):531–6.

CHAPTER 7

Integrin Antagonists and Angiogenesis

Shaker A. Mousa, Noureldien H.E. Darwish and Paul J. Davis

Contents

INTEGRINS

Integrins are a widely expressed family of cell adhesion receptor heterodimeric proteins that are essential to cell–cell and cell–extracellular matrix (ECM) protein interactions. Cell–cell communication and tissue structure require integrins. Integrins are composed of single α and β monomers. Most cells express several integrins, and the presence of both subunits is required to ensure normalcy of the interaction of integrins with the ECM and intracellularly with the cytoskeleton (Table 7.1).

Binding by integrins to their ligand proteins is cation-dependent. Specific ECM protein-integrin binding involves recognition by

Anti-Angiogenesis Strategies in Cancer Therapies
http://dx.doi.org/10.1016/B978-0-12-802576-5.00007-3

Table 7.1 αv Integrins: ligands and cellular and tissue distribution

αv Integrins	Ligands	Cellular and tissue distribution
αvβ1	Fn, Ln, Opn	Smooth muscle cells, fibroblasts, osteoclasts, tumor cells
αvβ3	ECM, Fg, Fn, MMP2, Opn, Tn, Tsp, Vn	Endothelial cells, smooth muscle cells, fibroblasts, osteoclasts, tumor cells, platelets, epithelial cells, leukocytes
αvβ5	Fg, Fn, Opn, Tsp, Vn	Endothelial cells, smooth muscle cells, fibroblasts, osteoclasts, tumor cells, platelets, epithelial cells, leukocytes
αvβ6	Fn, Fg, Tn, Vn	Epithelial cells, carcinoma cells
αvβ8	Vn	Melanoma, brain, kidney, ovary, placenta, uterus

Abbreviations: ECM, Extracellular matrix; Fg, fibrinogen; Fn, fibronectin; Ln, laminin; MMP, matrix metalloproteinase; Opn, osteopontin; Tn, tenascin; Tsp, thrombospondin; Vn, vitronectin.
Source: With permission of Springer: Mousa SA, Davis PJ. Angiogenesis modulations in health and disease, Integrin Antagonists and Angiogenesis, 2013, p. 120, [chapter 11].

integrins of specific amino acid sequences in their ligands. The most widely studied such sequence is Arg-Gly-Asp (RGD), found in 8 matrix proteins, including fibrinogen, vitronectin, fibronectin, thrombospondin, osteopontin, and von Willebrand factor (vWF) [1–3]. Additional integrins bind to ligands via non-RGD binding domains, for example, the Leu-Asp-Val (LDV) sequence within the connecting segment (CS-1) region of fibronectin and is recognized by α4β1 integrin. There are at least 8 α subunits and 14 β subunits [4–7]. The association of the known α and β monomers could theoretically result in more than 100 integrins, but the actual diversity is limited (Table 7.1).

INTEGRINS AND SIGNALING

The extracellular domain of integrins engages ECM ligands, and a cytoplasmic face of integrins relates to specific intracellular proteins, such as enzyme members of signal transducing kinase pathways. Binding by integrins of specific ECM proteins is not only important to cell adhesion, but they also support anchorage-dependent signaling within and between cells; such signaling is important to normal cell function and also underlies various pathological states (Fig. 7.1) [8–13]. An example of this is the activation of platelets that requires a conformational change in integrin αIIb/β3; the result is that the highly plastic integrin is converted into an activated fibrinogen receptor. The integrin-fibrinogen interaction results in activation of a panel of tyrosine kinases and phosphatases, as well as the attraction of a number of other signaling proteins. The latter are involved in the assembly of F-actin-rich cytoskeletal components at the cytoplasmic tails of monomeric αIIb and β3 in heterodimeric integrins [14]. Platelet function

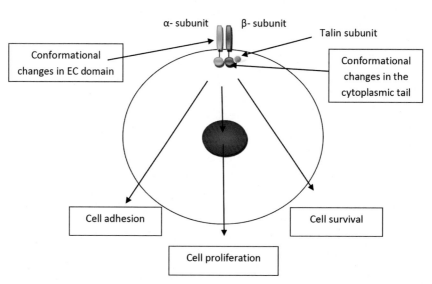

Figure 7.1 *Integrin activation.* External activating stimuli, such as selectin or integrin trigger intracellular signaling cascades. The activating signals lead to conformational changes in the integrin tails that facilitate the focal adhesion components (Talin). The conformational changes in the tail region will be extended to the extracellular domain resulting in structural rearrangements that will promote activation and increased affinity for the ligand.

is then regulated by coordinated signals emanating from cellular plasma membrane integrins and G-protein linked receptors [14].

The contributions of cytoplasmic tails of αIIb/β3 to intracellular signaling, apparently through physical interactions with signaling molecules and the cytoskeleton, have been documented by the induction of mutations in certain integrins [15]. Inhibition of the binding of fibrinogen to the extracellular domain of integrin αIIb/β3 can prevent local formation of platelet-rich coronary arterial thrombi after angioplasty in patients with coronary artery disease [16–18]. The inventory of proteins that are bound by cytoplasmic tails of αIIb/β3 is incomplete, but information that is available offers the possibility of developing pharmacologic inhibitors of integrin adhesion or signaling in ischemic organs or tissues [19]. The complexity of intracellular protein-integrin cytoplasmic tail interactions renders such a target more difficult to approach in drug design compared to single ECM protein-integrin interactions that occur with the extracellular domain of integrins.

CELL SURFACE MEMBRANE INTEGRINS AS POTENTIAL DRUG DISCOVERY TARGETS

Cell activation, migration, proliferation, differentiation, and other physiological processes depend on regularized, direct contact between cells and ECM. Cell–cell and cell–ECM require different families of cell adhesion molecules or multifunctional moieties that contribute to adhesion. Among these protein families are selectins, cadherins, integrins, and immunoglobulins. Cell adhesion molecules are of increasing pharmacologic interest [20,21].

The integrin superfamily represents a remarkable opportunity to develop targeted small molecule antagonists for therapeutic and diagnostic purposes because of the contributions that integrins make to normal cell and tissue function and to disease states.

β1 Integrins

Among the β monomer integrins, β1 has been shown to have an important role in cancers, especially in glioma biology. Expression of this integrin has been correlated with the invasive behavior of gliomas. $\beta1$ also contributes to the regulation of proliferation, differentiation, and migration of neural stem cells [22].

α2β1

The $\alpha2\beta1$ integrin (also known as GPIa/IIa, CD49b or VLA-2) was identified as an extracellular receptor for laminins and/or collagens. Recently, the $\alpha2\beta1$ integrin was found to be an important receptor for many molecules including matrix and nonmatrix molecules [23]. The $\alpha2\beta1$ is one of four "I domain" integrins, which are characterized by the presence of a highly conserved, extracellular, I domain. The I domain mediates specific binding of certain ligands, particularly, collagens [24].

$\alpha2\beta1$ is upregulated during vascular endothelial growth factor (VEGF)-induced angiogenesis in vivo and also in sprouting tips of neonatal blood vessels. This testifies to the important role of $\alpha2\beta1$ in angiogenesis, but the precise nature of the integrin's role is still incompletely understood. The earliest investigations into the functional role of $\alpha2\beta1$ in angiogenesis employed inhibitory antibodies during in vitro studies. Anti-$\alpha2$ inhibited tube and lumen formation by human umbilical vein endothelial cells in a 3D collagen matrix [24]. Senger and coworkers reported that inhibition of $\alpha2\beta1$ and $\alpha1\beta1$ in an in vivo model—using subcutaneous Matrigel plug angiogenesis assays in mice—was associated with a marked decrease in new vessel growth within the implanted plugs [25]. Thus, pharmacological inhibitors of $\alpha2\beta1$ may have useful anti-angiogenic effects [24].

α3β1

Integrin $\alpha3\beta1$ participates in angiogenesis and the pathogenesis of cancer. Hence, there is interest in developing antagonists of this protein or of specific receptors it bears. An $\alpha3\beta1$ integrin-binding site has been mapped to residues 190-201 (FQGVLQNVRFVF) of the N-terminal domain of thrombospondin-1 (TSP1), a protein that when secreted is anti-angiogenic. Suppression of expression of the *TSP1* gene is typical of cancer cells. Residues critical to biological activity of TSP1 are localized to a well-defined segment of the protein [26]. The NVR motif in residues 190–201 is required in the full-length TSP1 to enable recognition of the protein by the α3β1 integrin.

Integrin α3β1 has been shown to activate the signal transducing ERKs in some epithelial cells. While the signal transduction pathway activated by integrin α3 in the context of glioma cell migration and invasion is not clear, a recent study has demonstrated that integrin α3 can promote glioma cell invasiveness via ERK1/2 [22].

α5β1

Expression of fibronectin in ECM of provisional vascular matrices precedes permanent collagen expression. Fibronectin is involved in signaling to blood vessel cells and fibroblasts in the processes of blood coagulation and wound healing, of atherosclerosis and hypertension [27]. An isoform of fibronectin, the ED-B splice variant, is found in blood vessels in fetal and tumor tissues, but is not expressed by quiescent adult blood vessels [28]. Thus, this fibronectin variant appears to contribute to angiogenesis. Absence of fibronectin during embryonic development in animal models is fatal and associated with absence of the notochord and somites, as well as a defective vasculature [29]. Effective engagement of α5β1 integrin activates a nuclear factor κB (NFκB)–dependent gene expression program and importantly regulates the linked processes of angiogenesis and inflammation [30].

While several integrins are known to bind fibronectin, the association of α5β1 with fibronectin is regularly found [5]. It is not certain whether α5β1 plays a more important role in developmental blood vessel formation (vasculogenesis) or in blood vessel generation from existing vessels (angiogenesis). It is clear that fibronectin and integrin α5β1 do express coordinated function in angiogenesis [31,32], that is, the physical interaction of these two moieties is essential to angiogenesis. Integrin α5β1 overlaps functions of integrin αvβ3 in angiogenesis and these may be separate from roles played by αvβ5 [31,32]. Pharmacologic inhibition of α5β1 integrin thus might be useful in pathologic angiogenesis associated with cancer growth, inflammation, and certain ophthalmopathies [31,32].

Choroidal neovascularization is supported by upregulation of α5β1 [33]. Intraocular delivery of up to 12 mg/kg/day of a selective α5β1 inhibitor—3-(2-{1-alkyl-5-[(pyridin-2-ylamino)-methyl]-pyrrolidin-3-yloxy}-acetyl amino)-2-(alkyl amino)-propionic acid (JSM6427)—importantly suppressed choroidal neovascularization. Thus, α5β1 participates in choroidal neovascularization, and the integrin is a target [33] for small molecule inhibitors and α5β1 monoclonal antibody development [34,35].

β3 Integrins
αvβ3

Although the relationships between integrins and tumor cell cytoplasmic proteins are incompletely known, integrins have been shown in a variety of cells to complex with Src kinases, mitogen-activated protein kinase (MAPK, ERK), cytoskeletal proteins, growth factor receptors, Ras, NFκB, phosphatidylinositol 3-kinase (PI3-K), and protein kinase C [36]. This array of relationships is consistent with support by this integrin of tumor cell proliferation and anti-apoptosis defenses of tumor cells. Support of angiogenesis by this integrin is shown by the fact that inhibition of αvβ3 suppresses angiogenesis in various models and can result in tumor regression. The integrin also appears to be dormant on quiescent endothelial cells, but active under proangiogenic conditions.

The αv family of integrins associates with various integrin β subunits, and its interactions with diverse ECM proteins has a number of discrete functional implications (Table 7.1). cRGDfV is a selective inhibitor of αvβ3 and has been shown to be beneficial in experimental middle cerebral artery occlusion, apparently by a mechanism that is VEGF- and VEGF-receptor-dependent (Fig. 7.2) [37].

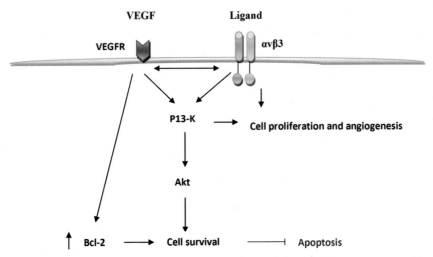

Figure 7.2 *Interactions between the integrin αvβ3 and VEGFR-2 may play a role in survival functions of VEGF.* Longer term anti-apoptotic effects of VEGF may involve upregulation of anti-apoptotic proteins, such as Bcl-2.

A variety of integrin antagonists are under development. Certain pyrazole and isoxazole analogs are inhibitors of αvβ3 and also have good selectivity for αIIb/β3. In HT29 cells, most of these analogs also demonstrated significant selectivity against αvβ6. Several newly developed compounds have also been shown to be effectively anti–angiogenic in a mouse corneal micro pocket model [38].

Integrin αvβ3 Antagonists Promote Tumor Regression by Inducing Apoptosis of Angiogenic Blood Vessels

A single intravascular injection of a cyclic peptide or monoclonal antibody antagonist of integrin αvβ3 disrupts ongoing angiogenesis on the chick chorioallantoic membrane (CAM) [39]. This anti-angiogenic effect is associated with prompt regression of a variety of human tumor cell xenografts transplanted onto this membrane. αvβ3 antagonists also suppress spontaneous pulmonary metastases of human melanoma cell xenografts [40–46]. In contrast, angiogenesis is promoted by (apparently αvβ3–negative) cancer cells resulting in the entry of dormant vascular cells into the cell cycle and expression of integrin $\alpha v\beta 3$. Pharmacological antagonists of this integrin induce apoptosis of tumor-associated, active vasculogenic cells, but do not affect preexisting adjacent or distant quiescent blood vessels [41]. Not unexpectedly, cultured human endothelial cells are resistant to proapoptotic pharmacological factors when they are attached to an immobilized $\alpha v\beta 3$ monoclonal antibody LM-609 [41]. The adhesion event appears to decrease endothelial cell expression of proapoptotic p53 and Bax, while increasing transcription of anti-apoptotic Bcl-2. Ligation of $\alpha v\beta 3$ is essential to the proliferation and metastatic potential of human cancer cells, as well as maturation of newly formed blood vessels [47–49]. In preclinical models, antibody or peptide antagonists of this integrin block tumor cell- and cytokine-induced angiogenesis. These inhibitors of $\alpha v\beta 3$ promote selective apoptosis of newly sprouting vessels. Thus, antagonists of integrin $\alpha v\beta 3$ have promise in management of disease processes critically dependent on angiogenesis [50].

Exploitation of $\alpha v\beta 3$ for Targeted Delivery of Viral or Pharmacologic Agents

IκB (dnIκB) is a naturally occurring protein inhibitor of NFκB-dependent signals transduction that is essential to TNF-α action. To selectively block NFκB and TNF-α actions in angiogenic endothelial cells, an $\alpha v\beta 3$ integrin-specific adenovirus encoding dominant negative IκB (dnIκB) was constructed [51]. An adenovirus targeted by RGD peptide to integrin $\alpha v\beta 3$ delivered dnIκB to dividing endothelial cells where dnIκB becomes functionally expressed. This led to complete abolition of TNF-α-induced upregulation of E-selectin, ICAM-1, VCAM-1, IL-6, IL-8, VEGF-A, and Tie-2 [51]. The targeted delivery process of dnIκB into endothelial cells may be useful in diseases, such as rheumatoid arthritis and inflammatory bowel disease. In these diseases, it is desirable to return activated NFκB to basal levels in the endothelium located, respectively, about inflamed joints or in the inflamed GI tract wall.

Most cancers express αvβ3 generously and such expression correlates with tumor progression. αvβ3 thus is an attractive target for drug design. Selective delivery of chemotherapeutic agents to αvβ3-positive metastatic cancer cells has already been reported, utilizing high affinity, small molecule αvβ3 ligands bound to the chemotherapeutic drugs [52–55].

Combination of αvβ3 Ligands and Tumor Imaging and Radiotherapy

Integrin αvβ3 is expressed at low levels on epithelial cells and mature endothelial cells, but is over-expressed on the activated endothelial cells of tumor neovasculature and on most tumor cells. The increased expression of integrin αvβ3 specifically during tumor growth, invasion, and metastasis presents an interesting molecular target for both early detection and treatment of rapidly growing solid tumors. A number of radiolabeled linear and cyclic RGD peptide ligands have been tested as integrin αvβ3 targeted radiotracers. Single photon emission computed tomography (SPECT) or positron emission tomography (PET) tumor imaging has been applied to tumor-bearing animal models. The first integrin αvβ3-targeted radiotracer under clinical diagnostic investigation in cancer patients is [^{18}F]Galacto-RGD. We emphasize here radiolabeled multimeric cyclic RGD peptides (dimers and tetramers) that are useful as radiotracers for tumor imaging by SPECT and PET and that have special requirements or features [56]. Such features are choice of radionuclide and bifunctional chelators, selection of targeting biomolecules, and factors that regulate affinity of αvβ3 for ligands, as well as different approaches for modification of radiotracer pharmacokinetics.

Radiotherapy is another approach to inhibition of tumor growth and modification of tumor-relevant vasculature [57]. A number of investigators have studied the combination of integrin antagonist cilengitide (EMD 121974) and ionizing radiation in cancer management. Expression and activation of αvβ3 integrin has been shown in endothelial and non-small cell lung cancer models to result from radiation exposure, and RGD-targeting of cilengitide has been found to have radiosensitizing properties that are proportional to the levels of integrin αvβ3 expression [57].

αv integrin monoclonal antibody (17E6) and a small molecule αvβ3, αvβ5 integrin inhibitor (EMD121974) have been reported to suppress tumor invasion and metastasis induced by the *CYR61* gene and to attenuate the metastatic potential of tumors growing within a preirradiated field [58]. Thus, αv integrin appears to be a therapeutic target in the prevention of metastasis in the setting of postradiation recurrences.

Antagonists of Integrins αvβ3 and αvβ5 Inhibit Angiogenesis

As indicated earlier, enhanced expression of αvβ3 during angiogenesis is critical to angiogenesis. Recent experimental evidence supports this notion. When angiogenesis is induced with purified cytokines in the chick CAM model, αvβ3 expression is increased fourfold within 72 h [40]. Applied topically in the CAM, monoclonal antibody to αvβ3, LM-609, inhibits angiogenesis, and other integrin antibodies do not affect new blood vessel formation [40]. In a model of tumor xenografts grown on the CAM surface, specific αvβ3 antagonists—LM-609 or cyclic RGD peptide inhibitors—downregulated blood vessel growth in tumor tissue. Preexisting vessels are unaffected by LM-609 [40]. These findings suggest that αvβ3 plays an important biological role in a late stage of blood vessel generation. Up to fivefold differences in tumor size or weight in various studies are reported between control tumors and anti-αvβ3-exposed lesions [40–43]. Injections of a cyclic RGD peptide, but not of an inactive control peptide, cause similar tumor regression. Few or no viable tumor cells remain in the anti-αvβ3 treated tumors when they are examined histologically. Treated tumors contain virtually no intact blood vessels [42].

Integrin αvβ3 antagonists have also been shown in preclinical studies to inhibit tumor growth in human skin. Brooks and colleagues established human neonatal foreskin grafts on SCID mice [41]. Human breast cancer growth in the skin grafts was fully suppressed or was significantly inhibited by αvβ3 antibody and control antibody was ineffective. There was at least 75% inhibition of angiogenesis in the tumors of LM-609 antibody-treated mice. αvβ3 antagonists also inhibit angiogenesis in ocular disease models. For example, integrin αvβ3 peptide antagonists inhibited retinal neovascularization in the oxygen-induced model of ischemic retinopathy (OIR) in the mouse [50].

A nonpeptidic antagonist of the αvβ3 and αvβ5 integrins, SB-267268, has been shown to limit angiogenesis in a murine model of retinopathy of prematurity (ROP). This action is a function of reduced expression of VEGF and a VEGF receptor [59]. Thus, nonpeptide antagonists of integrins αvβ3 and αvβ5 integrins are candidate therapies for ischemic retinal diseases.

Integrin αvβ3 Antagonists Versus Anti-αvβ3 and αvβ5

Mixtures of αvβ3 and αvβ5 inhibitors have been seen to be effective modalities in the treatment of disordered angiogenesis, since it was appreciated that these two αv-containing integrins participate in cytokine-induced angiogenesis [40,42]. Cyclic RGD pentapeptide mimics have been developed to affect these two integrins, including benzyl-substituted azabicycloalkane amino acids [60].

αvβ3 Ligands: Issues in the Development of αvβ3 Antagonists as Therapeutics

Preclinical investigations are in progress of a number of lead αvβ3 inhibitor products [61–65]. Several issues have slowed the development of these compounds. These problems include pharmacokinetics (PK) and pharmacodynamics (PD). The PK issues involve attempts to develop orally active compounds that have good bioavailability and satisfactory duration of half-lives. Optimizing dose is a problem because estimates of efficacy in animals or in vitro are not standardized and thus optimization of agents' efficacy/safety ratio (therapeutic index) has not been achieved [66].

Human serum albumin (HSA) binding of lead compounds is a major problem in drug discovery. Albumin-binding is a principal determinant of the availability of agents to their intended target and thus of drug efficacy. High HSA binding (> 97%) has been a major problem in the development of anti-integrin ($\alpha v \beta 3$, $\alpha v \beta 5$) compounds to date, despite their nanomolar binding affinities for their targets. Incorporation of polar groups into a lead compound may importantly decrease the affinity for HSA. Among the variety of anti-integrin compounds synthesized, 3-[5-[2-(5,6,7,8-tetrahydro[1,8]naphthyridin-2-yl)ethoxy]indol-1-yl]-3-[5-(N,N-dimethylaminomethyl)-3-pyridyl]propionic acid is an interesting model in that it has been shown to have satisfactory bioactivity, a sub-nanomolar affinity for both $\alpha v \beta 3$ and $\alpha v \beta 5$ and low HSA protein binding [34].

DIAGNOSTICS

Detection of tumor-related angiogenesis in vivo has been shown to be feasible by $\alpha v \beta 3$-targeted magnetic resonance imaging (MRI) [67–69] as has the imaging of cancer metastases with RGD peptide that is labeled with technetium-99m. Because of the selective increase in expression of $\alpha v \beta 3$ integrin in cancer cells and in rapidly dividing endothelial cells that are frequently associated with tumors, radiolabeled RGD peptides and peptidomimetics directed at $\alpha v \beta 3$ persist as attractive model compounds for tumor imaging [70].

Among various radiolabeled RGD peptides intended for tumor imaging [56], positron emitting ^{64}Cu-labeled pegylated dimeric RGD peptide radiotracer ^{64}Cu-DOTA-PEG-E[c(RGDyK)]$_2$ has emerged as a probe for lung cancer imaging [71]. The pegylated RGD peptide has demonstrated integrin $\alpha v \beta 3$ avidity, but the pegylation interestingly decreased integrin binding affinity of the agent compared to the unmodified RGD dimer. Rapid blood clearance and predominantly renal clearance of the compound were documented. In preclinical studies, there was minimal nonspecific tracer activity accumulation in normal lung tissue and in the heart. As a result, high–quality orthotopic lung cancer tumor images were enabled and there was clear demarcation of primary tumor and metastases in mediastinum and unaffected lung. In contrast, fluoro-deoxyglucose (FDG) scans on the same mice detected only the primary tumor because heart and normal lung uptakes produced high imaging backgrounds. ^{64}Cu-DOTA-PEG-E[c (RGDyK)]$_2$ is a PET tracer intended for integrin-positive tumor imaging [71] as mentioned earlier and the agent remains under development.

INTEGRIN–HORMONE CROSSTALK: INTEGRIN RECEPTOR-MEDIATED ACTIONS OF THYROID HORMONE

That thyroid hormone can act outside the cell nucleus has come from studies of mitochondrial responses to 3,5,3'-triiodo-L-thyronine (T$_3$) and from cell membrane or cytoplasmic actions of L-thyroxine (T$_4$) [72–78]. The description of a plasma membrane receptor for thyroid hormone on integrin αvβ3 [79–81] has provided insight into effects of the hormone on certain membrane ion pumps, such as the Na$^+$/H$^+$ anti-porter [74,82]. Such actions have also enabled descriptions of interfaces between the membrane thyroid hormone receptor and nuclear events that underlie important cellular or tissue processes, such as angiogenesis and proliferation of certain cancer cells [83–86].

The possible clinical utility of cellular events that are mediated by the membrane receptor for thyroid hormone may reside in inhibition of such effect(s) in the contexts of neovascularization or tumor cell growth. Indeed, we have shown that blocking the membrane receptor for iodothyronines with tetraiodothyroacetic acid (tetrac), a hormone-binding inhibitory analog that has no agonist activity at the receptor, can arrest growth of glioma cells and of human breast cancer cells in vitro [84]. Tetrac blocks the binding of T$_4$ and T$_3$ to αvβ3 and has anti-angiogenic and proapoptotic properties expressed via the integrin. We examined the possibility that tetrac action at the integrin may modulate vascular growth factor-induced angiogenesis in the absence of thyroid hormone. We have shown that tetrac blocks crosstalk between plasma-membrane vascular growth factor receptors and adjacent integrin $\alpha v \beta 3$ and downregulates expression of certain vascular growth factor genes [87]. Tetrac is a useful probe to screen for the participation of the integrin receptor in actions of thyroid hormone.

Integrin $\alpha v \beta 3$ bears a receptor for tetrac near the RGD recognition site of the protein. The hormone receptor is anatomically and, in large measure, functionally separate from the RGD site that conditions the binding by the integrin of certain ECM proteins [80]. The intact integrin is structurally very plastic [88]. Its conformational changes in response to ligand-binding may underlie its ability to transduce cell surface signals from a variety of extracellular matrix proteins or small molecules into discrete intracellular messages, as well as its ability to expose new extracellular domain surfaces for interactions with ligands. The thyroid hormone signal at the integrin is transduced via the intracellular (cytoplasmic) domain or tail of the protein into MAPK activity via phospholipase C and protein kinase C (PKC) [89]. MAPK (ERK1/2) activation is associated with increased Na^+/H^+ anti-porter (exchanger) activity locally in the plasma membrane as a function of thyroid hormone concentration. We have speculated that hormone effects on other ion pumps at the cell surface, for example, Ca^{2+}-ATPase and Na,K-ATPase, also relate to MAPK and PKC activation [82]. The complex process of angiogenesis is also regulated by thyroid hormone and tetrac at the plasma membrane, as documented in the CAM assay or by human endothelial cells in a sprouting assay [83]. This is another integrin-dependent mechanism that involves MAPK activation. Downstream of the integrin and signaling kianses, thyroid hormone's initiation of angiogenesis involves elaboration of basic fibroblast growth factor (b-FGF; FGF2) [83] and enhanced endothelial mobility in response to specific protein cures [83]. It is possible that desirable neovascularization can be promoted with local application of thyroid hormone analogs, for example, in wound-healing, or that undesirable angiogenesis, such as that which supports tumor growth, can be antagonized in part with tetrac. The broadly based angiogenesis regulation capability of tetrac formulations has been shown in CAM studies in which T_4 and T_3 are absent; here, tetrac or Nanotetrac inhibit proangiogenic actions of VEGF, FGF2, platelet derived growth factor, and small molecule stimulators of new blood vessel formation [90,91]. Nanotetrac also downregulates transcription of angiogenesis-relevant *VEGF-A* and *EGFR* genes.

Thyroid hormone as T_4 also enhances in vitro proliferation of certain tumor cells [80], including glioma cell lines [86]. In a clinical corollary, Hercbergs and coworkers conducted a prospective study of medically induced hypothyroidism in patients with far advanced glioblastoma multiforme [92]. An important survival benefit was achieved in patients with mild hypothyroidism. Human breast cancer MCF-7 cells were shown by us a decade ago to proliferate in response to T_4 by a tetrac-sensitive mechanism [85]. In another clinical corollary, Cristofanilli and coworkers showed that hypothyroid women who developed breast cancer did so later in life than matched euthyroid controls. In addition, the cancers were smaller and less aggressive at the time of diagnosis than cancers in euthyroid control breast cancer patients. We conclude that thyroid hormone has a trophic action on in vitro models of brain tumor and breast cancer that appears to be reflected in clinical disease [92,93].

CONCLUSIONS

Inhibition of $\alpha v \beta 3$-proangiogenic ligand interaction by integrin antibody or peptide antagonists results in endothelial cell apoptosis and inhibits angiogenesis. Such observations encourage further study of the complex regulation by this integrin of angiogenesis and the search for novel therapeutic strategies to disrupt the contributions to angiogenesis-related diseases that are mediated by integrin $\alpha v \beta 3$.

Combinations of chemotherapy or radiotherapy with integrin antagonists appear in preclinical studies to be effective anti-cancer interventions. Radiotherapy has been shown to enhance expression of $\alpha v\beta 3$ by endothelial cells, an observation that suggests that interventional radiation can sensitize cells to the actions of pharmacological inhibitors of $\alpha v\beta 3$. Drug resistance mechanisms may also be opposed by $\alpha v\beta 3$ inhibitors when combined with other anti-angiogenesis strategies.

REFERENCES

[1] Hwang DS, Sim SB, Cha HJ. Cell adhesion biomaterial based on mussel adhesive protein fused with RGD peptide. Biomaterials 2007;28(28):4039–46.

[2] Ruoslahti E. The RGD story: a personal account. Matrix Biol 2003;22(6):459–65.

[3] Ruoslahti E, Pierschbacher MD. New perspectives in cell adhesion: RGD and integrins. Science 1987;238(4826):491–7.

[4] Ruoslahti E, Pierschbacher MD. Arg-Gly-Asp: a versatile cell recognition signal. Cell 1986;44(4):517–8.

[5] Hynes RO. Integrins: versatility, modulation, and signaling in cell adhesion. Cell 1992;69(1):11–25.

[6] Cox D, Aoki T, Seki J, Motoyama Y, Yoshida K. The pharmacology of the integrins. Med Res Rev 1994;14(2):195–228.

[7] Albelda SM, Buck CA. Integrins and other cell adhesion molecules. FASEB J 1990;4(11):2868–80.

[8] Wickham TJ, Mathias P, Cheresh DA, Nemerow GR. Integrins $\alpha v\beta 3$ and $\alpha v\beta 5$ promote adenovirus internalization but not virus attachment. Cell 1993;73(2):309–19.

[9] Guadagno TM, Ohtsubo M, Roberts JM, Assoian RK. A link between cyclin A expression and adhesion-dependent cell cycle progression. Science 1993;262(5139):1572–5.

[10] Juliano RL, Haskill S. Signal transduction from the extracellular matrix. J Cell Biol 1993;120(3):577–85.

[11] Kornberg LJ, Earp HS, Turner CE, Prockop C, Juliano RL. Signal transduction by integrins: increased protein tyrosine phosphorylation caused by clustering of beta 1 integrins. Proc Natl Acad Sci USA 1991;88(19):8392–6.

[12] Kornberg L, Earp HS, Parsons JT, Schaller M, Juliano RL. Cell adhesion or integrin clustering increases phosphorylation of a focal adhesion-associated tyrosine kinase. J Biol Chem 1992;267(33):23439–42.

[13] Guan JL, Shalloway D. Regulation of focal adhesion-associated protein tyrosine kinase by both cellular adhesion and oncogenic transformation. Nature 1992;358(6388):690–2.

[14] Pelletier AJ, Bodary SC, Levinson AD. Signal transduction by the platelet integrin alpha IIb beta 3: induction of calcium oscillations required for protein-tyrosine phosphorylation and ligand-induced spreading of stably transfected cells. Mol Biol Cell 1992;3(9):989–98.

[15] Vinogradova O, Velyvis A, Velyviene A, Hu B, Haas T, Plow E, Qin J. A structural mechanism of integrin αIIbβ3 "inside-out" activation as regulated by its cytoplasmic face. Cell 2002;110(5):587–97.

[16] Topol EJ, Califf RM, Weisman HF, Ellis SG, Tcheng JE, Worley S, Ivanhoe R, George BS, Fintel D, Weston M, et al. Randomised trial of coronary intervention with antibody against platelet IIb/IIIa integrin for reduction of clinical restenosis: results at six months. The EPIC investigators. Lancet 1994;343(8902):881–6.

[17] The EPIC Investigators. Use of a monoclonal antibody directed against the platelet glycoprotein IIb/IIIa receptor in high-risk coronary angioplasty. N Engl J Med 1994;330(14):956–61.

[18] Mousa SA. Antiplatelet therapies: from aspirin to GPIIb/IIIa-receptor antagonists and beyond. Drug Discov Today 1999;4(12):552–61.

[19] Ma YQ, Qin J, Plow EF. Platelet integrin αIIbβ3: activation mechanisms. J Thromb Haemost 2007;5(7):1345–52.

[20] Staunton DE, Marlin SD, Stratowa C, Dustin ML, Springer TA. Primary structure of ICAM-1 demonstrates interaction between members of the immunoglobulin and integrin supergene families. Cell 1988;52(6): 925–33.

[21] Romo GM, Dong J-F, Schade AJ, Gardiner EE, Kansas GS, Li CQ, McIntire LV, Berndt MC, López JA. The glycoprotein Ib-IX-V complex is a platelet counterreceptor for P-selectin. J Exp Med 1999;190(6):803–14.

[22] Nakada M, Nambu E, Furuyama N, Yoshida Y, Takino T, Hayashi Y, Sato H, Sai Y, Tsuji T, Miyamoto KI, Hirao A, Hamada JI. Integrin α3 is overexpressed in glioma stem-like cells and promotes invasion. Br J Cancer 2013;108(12):2516–24.

[23] Habart D, Cheli Y, Nugent DJ, Ruggeri ZM, Kunicki TJ. Conditional knockout of integrin α2β1 in murine megakaryocytes leads to reduced mean platelet volume. PLoS One 2013;8(1):e55094.

[24] Madamanchi A, Santoro SA, Zutter MM. α2β1 Integrin. Adv Exp Med Biol 2014;819:41–60.

[25] Senger DR, Claffey KP, Benes JE, Perruzzi CA, Sergiou AP, Detmar M. Angiogenesis promoted by vascular endothelial growth factor: regulation

through $\alpha1\beta1$ and $\alpha2\beta1$ integrins. Proc Natl Acad Sci USA 1997; 94(25):13612–7.

[26] Furrer J, Luy B, Basrur V, Roberts DD, Barchi JJ Jr. Conformational analysis of an $\alpha3\beta1$ integrin-binding peptide from thrombospondin-1: implications for antiangiogenic drug design. J Med Chem 2006;49(21): 6324–33.

[27] Magnusson MK, Mosher DF. Fibronectin: structure, assembly, and cardio-vascular implications. Arterioscler Thromb Vasc Biol 1998;18(9):1363–70.

[28] Neri D, Carnemolla B, Nissim A, Leprini A, Querze G, Balza E, Pini A, Tarli L, Halin C, Neri P, Zardi L, Winter G. Targeting by affinity-matured recombinant antibody fragments of an angiogenesis associated fibronectin isoform. Nat Biotechnol 1997;15(12):1271–5.

[29] George EL, Georges-Labouesse EN, Patel-King RS, Rayburn H, Hynes RO. Defects in mesoderm, neural tube and vascular development in mouse embryos lacking fibronectin. Development 1993;119(4):1079–91.

[30] Klein S, de Fougerolles AR, Blaikie P, Khan L, Pepe A, Green CD, Koteliansky V, Giancotti FG. $\alpha5\beta1$ integrin activates an NF-κB-dependent program of gene expression important for angiogenesis and inflammation. Mol Cell Biol 2002;22(16):5912–22.

[31] Varner JA, Mousa SA. Antagonists of vascular cell integrin alpha 5 beta 1 inhibit angiogenesis. Circulation 1998;98(17):795.

[32] Mousa S, Mohamed S, Smallheer J, Jadhav P, Varner J. Anti-angiogene-sis efficacy of small molecule $\alpha5\beta1$ integrin antagonists, SJ749. Blood 1999;94(10):S1.

[33] Umeda N, Kachi S, Akiyama H, Zahn G, Vossmeyer D, Stragies R, Cam-pochiaro PA. Suppression and regression of choroidal neovascularization by systemic administration of an $\alpha5\beta1$ integrin antagonist. Mol Pharma-col 2006;69(6):1820–8.

[34] Raboisson P, Manthey CL, Chaikin M, Lattanze J, Crysler C, Leonard K, Pan W, Tomczuk BE, Marugan JJ. Novel potent and selective $\alpha v\beta3/\alpha v\beta5$ integrin dual antagonists with reduced binding affinity for human serum albumin. Eur J Med Chem 2006;41(7):847–61.

[35] Benfatti F, Cardillo G, Fabbroni S, Galzerano P, Gentilucci L, Juris R, Tolomelli A, Baiula M, Sparta A, Spampinato S. Synthesis and biologi-cal evaluation of non-peptide $\alpha v\beta3/\alpha5\beta1$ integrin dual antagonists containing 5,6-dihydropyridin-2-one scaffolds. Bioorg Med Chem 2007;15(23):7380–90.

[36] Pechkovsky DV, Scaffidi AK, Hackett TL, Ballard J, Shaheen F, Thompson PJ, Thannickal VJ, Knight DA. Transforming growth factor $\beta1$ induces $\alpha v\beta3$ integrin expression in human lung fibroblasts via a

β3 integrin-, c-Src-, and p38 MAPK-dependent pathway. J Biol Chem 2008;283(19):12898–908.

[37] Shimamura N, Matchett G, Yatsushige H, Calvert JW, Ohkuma H, Zhang J. Inhibition of integrin αvβ3 ameliorates focal cerebral ischemic damage in the rat middle cerebral artery occlusion model. Stroke 2006;37(7):1902–9.

[38] Penning TD, Khilevich A, Chen BB, Russell MA, Boys ML, Wang Y, Duffin T, Engleman VW, Finn MB, Freeman SK, Hanneke ML, Keene JL, Klover JA, Nickols GA, Nickols MA, Rader RK, Settle SL, Shannon KE, Steininger CN, Westlin MM, Westlin WF. Synthesis of pyrazoles and isoxazoles as potent αvβ3 receptor antagonists. Bioorg Med Chem Lett 2006;16(12):3156–61.

[39] Brooks PC, Clark RA, Cheresh DA. Requirement of vascular integrin alpha v beta 3 for angiogenesis. Science 1994;264(5158):569–71.

[40] Sanders LC, Felding-Habermann B, Mueller BM, Cheresh DA. Role of alpha V integrins and vitronectin in human melanoma cell growth. Cold Spring Harb Symp Quant Biol 1992;57:233–40.

[41] Brooks PC, Strömblad S, Klemke R, Visscher D, Sarkar FH, Cheresh DA. Antiintegrin alpha v beta 3 blocks human breast cancer growth and angiogenesis in human skin. J Clin Invest 1995;96(4):1815.

[42] Hieken TJ, Farolan M, Ronan SG, Shilkaitis A, Wild L, Das Gupta TK. Beta3 integrin expression in melanoma predicts subsequent metastasis. J Surg Res 1996;63(1):169–73.

[43] Albelda SM, Mette SA, Elder DE, Stewart R, Damjanovich L, Herlyn M, Buck CA. Integrin distribution in malignant melanoma: association of the β 3 subunit with tumor progression. Cancer Res 1990;50(20):6757–64.

[44] Nip J, Brodt P. The role of the integrin vitronectin receptor, alpha v beta 3 in melanoma metastasis. Cancer Metastasis Rev 1995;14(3):241–52.

[45] Max R, Gerritsen RR, Nooijen PT, Goodman SL, Sutter A, Keilholz U, Ruiter DJ, De Waal RM. Immunohistochemical analysis of integrin αvβ3 expression on tumor-associated vessels of human carcinomas. Int J Cancer 1997;71(3):320–4.

[46] Clark R, Tonnesen M, Gailit J. Transient functional expression of alpha-Vbeta 3 on vascular cells during wound repair. Am J Pathol 1996;148:1407–21.

[47] Eliceiri B, Klemke R, Stromblad S, Cheresh D. Integrin αVβ3 requirement for sustained mitogenactivated protein kinase activated protein kinase activity during angiogenesis. J Cell Biol 1999;14:1255–63.

[48] Friedlander M, Brooks PC, Shaffer RW, Kincaid CM, Varner JA, Cheresh DA. Definition of two angiogenic pathways by distinct αv integrins. Science 1995;270(5241):1500–2.

[49] Eliceiri BP, Cheresh DA. The role of αv integrins during angiogenesis: insights into potential mechanisms of action and clinical development. J Clin Invest 1999;103(9):1227–30.

[50] Luna J, Tobe T, Mousa SA, Reilly TM, Campochiaro PA. Antagonists of integrin alpha v beta 3 inhibit retinal neovascularization in a murine model. Lab Invest 1996;75(4):563–73.

[51] Ogawara K-i, Kucdo J, Oosterhuis K, Kroesen B, Rots MG, Trautwein C, Kimura T, Haisma HJ, Molema G. Functional inhibition of NF-κB signal transduction in αvβ3 integrin expressing endothelial cells by using RGD-PEG-modified adenovirus with a mutant IκB gene. Arthritis Res Ther 2006;8(1):R32.

[52] Curnis F, Sacchi A, Gasparri A, Longhi R, Bachi A, Doglioni C, Bordignon C, Traversari C, Rizzardi G-P, Corti A. Isoaspartate-glycine-arginine: a new tumor vasculature–targeting motif. Cancer Res 2008;68(17): 7073–82.

[53] Zhao H, Wang J-C, Sun Q-S, Luo C-L, Zhang Q. RGD-based strategies for improving antitumor activity of paclitaxel-loaded liposomes in nude mice xenografted with human ovarian cancer. J Drug Target 2009;17(1):10–8.

[54] Garanger E, Boturyn D, Dumy P. Tumor targeting with RGD peptide ligands-design of new molecular conjugates for imaging and therapy of cancers. Anticancer Agents Med Chem 2007;7(5):552–8.

[55] Dayam R, Aiello F, Deng J, Wu Y, Garofalo A, Chen X, Neamati N. Discovery of small molecule integrin αvβ3 antagonists as novel anticancer agents. J Med Chem 2006;49(15):4526–34.

[56] Wu Z, Li ZB, Chen K, Cai W, He L, Chin FT, Li F, Chen X. microPET of tumor integrin αvβ3 expression using ^{18}F-labeled PEGylated tetrameric RGD peptide (^{18}F-FPRGD$_4$). J Nucl Med 2007;48(9):1536–44.

[57] Albert JM, Cao C, Geng L, Leavitt L, Hallahan DE, Lu B. Integrin αvβ3 antagonist Cilengitide enhances efficacy of radiotherapy in endothelial cell and non-small-cell lung cancer models. Int J Radiat Oncol Biol Phys 2006;65(5):1536–43.

[58] Monnier Y, Farmer P, Bieler G, Imaizumi N, Sengstag T, Alghisi GC, Stehle JC, Ciarloni L, Andrejevic-Blant S, Moeckli R, Mirimanoff RO, Goodman SL, Delorenzi M, Ruegg C. CYR61 and αvβ5 integrin cooperate to

promote invasion and metastasis of tumors growing in preirradiated stroma. Cancer Res 2008;68(18):7323–31.

[59] Wilkinson-Berka JL, Jones D, Taylor G, Jaworski K, Kelly DJ, Ludbrook SB, Willette RN, Kumar S, Gilbert RE. SB-267268, a nonpeptidic antagonist of αvβ3 and αvβ5 integrins, reduces angiogenesis and VEGF expression in a mouse model of retinopathy of prematurity. Invest Ophthalmol Vis Sci 2006;47(4):1600–5.

[60] Arosio D, Belvisi L, Colombo L, Colombo M, Invernizzi D, Manzoni L, Potenza D, Serra M, Castorina M, Pisano C, Scolastico C. A potent integrin antagonist from a small library of cyclic RGD pentapeptide mimics including benzyl-substituted azabicycloalkane amino acids. ChemMedChem 2008;3(10):1589–603.

[61] Keenan RM, Miller WH, Kwon C, Ali FE, Callahan JF, Calvo RR, Hwang SM, Kopple KD, Peishoff CE, Samanen JM, Wong AS, Yuan CK, Huffman WF. Discovery of potent nonpeptide vitronectin receptor (αvβ3) antagonists. J Med Chem 1997;40(15):2289–92.

[62] Corbett JW, Graciani NR, Mousa SA, DeGrado WF. Solid-phase synthesis of a selective αvβ3 integrin antagonist library. Bioorg Med Chem Lett 1997;7(11):1371–6.

[63] Knolle J, Baron R, Breipohl G, Broto P, Gadek T, Gourvest JF, Hammonds GR, Peyman A, Scheunemann KH, Stilz HU. Design and synthesis of potent and selective peptidomimetic vitronectin receptor antagonists. Peptides Frontiers of Peptide Science. Netherlands: Springer; 2002. p. 181–182.

[64] Kerr JS, Wexler R, Mousa S, Robinson C, Wexler E, Mohamed S, Voss M, Devenny J, Czerniak P, Gudzelak A Jr. Novel small molecule alpha v integrin antagonists: comparative anti-cancer efficacy with known angiogenesis inhibitors. Anticancer Res 1998;19(2A):959–68.

[65] Mousa SA, Lorelli W, Mohamed S, Batt DG, Jadhav PK, Reilly TM. αvβ3 integrin binding affinity and specificity of SM256 in various species. J Cardiovasc Pharmacol 1999;33(4):641–6.

[66] Arap W, Pasqualini R, Ruoslahti E. Cancer treatment by targeted drug delivery to tumor vasculature in a mouse model. Science 1998;279(5349): 377–80.

[67] Sipkins DA, Cheresh DA, Kazemi MR, Nevin LM, Bednarski MD, Li KC. Detection of tumor angiogenesis in vivo by alphaVbeta3-targeted magnetic resonance imaging. Nat Med 1998;4(5):623–6.

[68] Sivolapenko GB, Skarlos D, Pectasides D, Stathopoulou E, Milonakis A, Sirmalis G, Stuttle A, Courtenay-Luck NS, Konstantinides K, Epenetos

AA. Imaging of metastatic melanoma utilising a technetium-99m labelled RGD-containing synthetic peptide. Eur J Nucl Med 1998;25(10):1383–9.

[69] Haubner R, Wester HJ, Reuning U, Senekowitsch-Schmidtke R, Diefenbach B, Kessler H, Stocklin G, Schwaiger M. Radiolabeled $\alpha v \beta 3$ integrin antagonists: a new class of tracers for tumor targeting. J Nucl Med 1999;40(6):1061–71.

[70] Dijkgraaf I, Kruijtzer JA, Frielink C, Soede AC, Hilbers HW, Oyen WJ, Corstens FH, Liskamp RM, Boerman OC. Synthesis and biological evaluation of potent $\alpha v \beta 3$-integrin receptor antagonists. Nucl Med Biol 2006;33(8):953–61.

[71] Chen X, Sievers E, Hou Y, Park R, Tohme M, Bart R, Bremner R, Bading JR, Conti PS. Integrin $\alpha v \beta 3$-targeted imaging of lung cancer. Neoplasia 2005;7(3):271–9.

[72] Huang CJ, Geller HM, Green WL, Craelius W. Acute effects of thyroid hormone analogs on sodium currents in neonatal rat myocytes. J Mol Cell Cardiol 1999;31(4):881–93.

[73] Sakaguchi Y, Cui G, Sen L. Acute effects of thyroid hormone on inward rectifier potassium channel currents in guinea pig ventricular myocytes. Endocrinology 1996;137(11):4744–51.

[74] Incerpi S, Luly P, De Vito P, Farias RN. Short-term effects of thyroid hormones on the Na/H antiport in L-6 myoblasts: high molecular specificity for 3,3',5-triiodo-L-thyronine. Endocrinology 1999;140(2):683–9.

[75] Ashizawa K, Cheng SY. Regulation of thyroid hormone receptor-mediated transcription by a cytosol protein. Proc Natl Acad Sci USA 1992;89(19):9277–81.

[76] Vie MP, Evrard C, Osty J, Breton-Gilet A, Blanchet P, Pomerance M, Rouget P, Francon J, Blondeau JP. Purification, molecular cloning, and functional expression of the human nicodinamide-adenine dinucleotide phosphate-regulated thyroid hormone-binding protein. Mol Endocrinol 1997;11(11):1728–36.

[77] Wrutniak-Cabello C, Casas F, Cabello G. Thyroid hormone action in mitochondria. J Mol Endocrinol 2001;26(1):67–77.

[78] Silvestri E, Schiavo L, Lombardi A, Goglia F. Thyroid hormones as molecular determinants of thermogenesis. Acta Physiol Scand 2005;184(4): 265–83.

[79] Bergh JJ, Lin HY, Lansing L, Mohamed SN, Davis FB, Mousa S, Davis PJ. Integrin $\alpha v \beta 3$ contains a cell surface receptor site for thyroid hormone that is linked to activation of mitogen-activated protein kinase and induction of angiogenesis. Endocrinology 2005;146(7):2864–71.

[80] Davis PJ, Davis FB, Cody V. Membrane receptors mediating thyroid hormone action. Trends Endocrinol Metab 2005;16(9):429–35.

[81] Mousa SA, O'Connor L, Davis FB, Davis PJ. Proangiogenesis action of the thyroid hormone analog 3,5-diiodothyropropionic acid (DITPA) is initiated at the cell surface and is integrin mediated. Endocrinology 2006;147(4):1602–7.

[82] D'Arezzo S, Incerpi S, Davis FB, Acconcia F, Marino M, Farias RN, Davis PJ. Rapid nongenomic effects of 3,5,3'-triiodo-L-thyronine on the intracellular pH of L-6 myoblasts are mediated by intracellular calcium mobilization and kinase pathways. Endocrinology 2004;145(12):5694–703.

[83] Davis FB, Mousa SA, O'Connor L, Mohamed S, Lin HY, Cao HJ, Davis PJ. Proangiogenic action of thyroid hormone is fibroblast growth factor-dependent and is initiated at the cell surface. Circ Res 2004;94(11):1500–6.

[84] Mousa SA, O'Connor LJ, Bergh JJ, Davis FB, Scanlan TS, Davis PJ. The proangiogenic action of thyroid hormone analogue GC-1 is initiated at an integrin. J Cardiovasc Pharmacol 2005;46(3):356–60.

[85] Tang HY, Lin HY, Zhang S, Davis FB, Davis PJ. Thyroid hormone causes mitogen-activated protein kinase-dependent phosphorylation of the nuclear estrogen receptor. Endocrinology 2004;145(7):3265–72.

[86] Davis FB, Tang HY, Shih A, Keating T, Lansing L, Hercbergs A, Fenstermaker RA, Mousa A, Mousa SA, Davis PJ, Lin HY. Acting via a cell surface receptor, thyroid hormone is a growth factor for glioma cells. Cancer Res 2006;66(14):7270–5.

[87] Mousa SA, Bergh JJ, Dier E, Rebbaa A, O'Connor LJ, Yalcin M, Aljada A, Dyskin E, Davis FB, Lin HY, Davis PJ. Tetraiodothyroacetic acid, a small molecule integrin ligand, blocks angiogenesis induced by vascular endothelial growth factor and basic fibroblast growth factor. Angiogenesis 2008;11(2):183–90.

[88] Xiong JP, Stehle T, Diefenbach B, Zhang R, Dunker R, Scott DL, Joachimiak A, Goodman SL, Arnaout MA. Crystal structure of the extracellular segment of integrin $\alpha v \beta 3$. Science 2001;294(5541):339–45.

[89] Lin HY, Davis FB, Gordinier JK, Martino LJ, Davis PJ. Thyroid hormone induces activation of mitogen-activated protein kinase in cultured cells. Am J Physiol Cell Physiol 1999;276(5):C1014–24.

[90] Mousa SA, Lin HY, Tang HY, Hercbergs A, Luidens MK, Davis PJ. Modulation of angiogenesis by thyroid hormone and hormone analogues: implications for cancer management. Angiogenesis 2014;17(3):463–9.

[91] Davis PJ, Sudha T, Lin HY, Mousa SA. Thyroid hormone, hormone analogs, and angiogenesis. Compr Physiol 2015;6(1):353–62.

[92] Hercbergs AA, Goyal LK, Suh JH, Lee S, Reddy CA, Cohen BH, Stevens GH, Reddy SK, Peereboom DM, Elson PJ, Gupta MK, Barnett GH. Propylthiouracil-induced chemical hypothyroidism with high-dose tamoxifen prolongs survival in recurrent high grade glioma: a phase I/II study. Anticancer Res 2003;23(1B):617–26.

[93] Cristofanilli M, Yamamura Y, Kau SW, Bevers T, Strom S, Patangan M, Hsu L, Krishnamurthy S, Theriault RL, Hortobagyi GN. Thyroid hormone and breast carcinoma. Primary hypothyroidism is associated with a reduced incidence of primary breast carcinoma. Cancer 2005;103(6):1122–8.

CHAPTER 8

Tyrosine Kinase Inhibitors and Angiogenesis

Paul J. Davis and Shaker A. Mousa

Contents

Introduction

The principal vascular growth factor proteins are vascular endothelial growth factor (VEGF), basic fibroblast growth factor (bFGF), platelet-derived growth factor (PDGF), and epidermal growth factor (EGF). Each of these angiogenesis-stimulating proteins has a cell surface receptor, for example, VEGFR, bFGFR, PDGFR, and EGFR, bearing one or more tyrosine kinases. Phosphorylation of a tyrosine activates such receptors, thus initiating the intracellular proangiogenesis signaling pathway. For about thirty years, pharmaceutical engineering has generated a substantial number of tyrosine kinase inhibitors (TKIs) intended to block angiogenesis that is tumor-related and, in the example of EGF and EGFR, to act directly on tumor cells. A number of TKIs have been approved by the US Food and Drug Administration (FDA) for clinical use against specific cancers.

Anti-Angiogenesis Strategies in Cancer Therapies
http://dx.doi.org/10.1016/B978-0-12-802576-5.00008-5

Examples of Specific TKIs
Sunitinib

Sunitinib is a small molecule TKI that prevents activation of vascular growth factor PDGFRα, hPDGFRβ, VEGFR-1, VEGFR-2, VEGFR-3, and other cell surface receptors relevant to cancer cell biology [1,2]. Interference with activation of these receptors downregulates a panel of intracellular signaling pathways. Sunitinib has been approved for the treatment of several solid tumors, including renal cell carcinoma, gastrointestinal tract stromal tumors, and advanced pancreatic neuroendocrine cancer.

Sorafenib

Sorafenib acts on vascular growth factor receptors VEGFR-1, VEGFR-2, VEGFR-3, and PDGFRβ [3] and their subservient signal transduction pathways. The agent has been approved for clinical use in advanced renal cell carcinoma and advanced, that is, inoperable, hepatocellular carcinoma.

Sunitinib and sorafenib are recognized to have the side effect of inducing thyroid gland destruction and hypothyroidism. This is an important observation because of the complex proangiogenic properties of thyroid hormone [4,5] that affect multiple discrete molecular mechanisms by which new blood vessels are generated. These actions of thyroid hormone are initiated at a plasma membrane receptor on integrin $\alpha v\beta 3$ [6,7] and enhance crosstalk between the integrin and adjacent vascular growth factor receptors and, downstream within the cell, the transcription of a variety of angiogenesis-related genes.

Vandetinib

Vandetinib binds to VEGF and EGF receptors, serving to inactivate the kinase, and influencing thereby a set of angiogenesis-relevant signaling systems. The agent has been approved for clinical use against advanced medullary carcinoma of the thyroid gland [8,9].

Pazopanib

Pazopanib serves to inhibit the tyrosine kinase activity of receptors VEGFR-1, VEGFR-2, VEGFR-3, PDGFα, PDGFβ, FGFR-1 and FGFR-3 [10]. The agent has been approved for clinical application in patients with renal cell carcinoma.

Axitinib

Axitinib targets VEGFR-1, VEGFR-2, VEGFR-3, and PDGFR [10]. It has been approved for use in patients with advanced renal cell carcinoma. Overall survival (OS) was not improved in axitinib-treated patients compared to a sorafenib cohort. Progression-free survival (PFS) analysis is complex in this comparison [10].

Nintedanib

Nintedanib is a triple angiogenesis pathway agent that affects the VEGF, FGF, and PDGFR pathways [11] and has been studied clinically in Europe. Small positive benefits have been obtained in early trials versus lung cancer in terms of PFS and as little as 2 months' improvement in OS.

Impact of Angiogenesis-Active TKIs on Clinical Outcomes

Most of these agents have had modest, favorable effects on the clinical courses of the specific tumors to which they have been applied. Meta-analysis of the effectiveness of groups of multitargeted anti-angiogenic TKIs has demonstrated little or no superiority to chemotherapy, alone, in terms of OS and PFS [12], despite some improvement for short-term in tumor status (overall response rate, ORR). There is increased pharmacologic interest currently in VEGFR-2 inhibition because of the multifactorial action of this particular receptor on endothelial cell proliferation, motility, and differentiation [13].

The limited effects of TKIs have been attributed to the complexity of regulation of angiogenesis that is vested in tumor cells and the fact that no one agent affects VEGFRs, FGFRs, PDGFRs, and EGFR; thus, escape mechanisms exist for tumor cells exposed to agents that primarily affect VEGF/VEGFR. Further, multiple TKI resistance pathways exist [14] and may be activated in tumor cells, for example, at EGFR [15]. Resistance to TKIs in cancer cells may also be based in tumor cell export mechanisms, that is, the plasma membrane ATP-binding cassette (ABC) transporter that rids cells of a variety of drugs [16].

Another adverse factor for TKIs is the several patterns of cardiotoxicity that have been described [17] and that can limit the duration of patient exposure.

Conclusions

The tyrosine kinase activity of the principal cell surface vascular growth factor receptors is an attractive target in anti-cancer pharmacology. Inhibition of this activity by TKI drugs impairs specific vascular growth factor signaling. The redundancy of such growth factors—VEGF, bFGF, PDGF, and EGF—and their receptors offers cancers a set of signaling options when only one or a small number of growth factors or growth factor isoform receptors is affected by a TKI. That is, the anti-angiogenic/anti-cancer actions of currently available TKIs may be limited in extent or time or both. Development continues of TKI designs with a broader base of receptor targets and this is desirable. Other factors that limit the use of these agents are the development of drug resistance and the side effect profiles of the drugs.

Additional strategies for the improvement of anti-angiogenic responses to TKIs are the possibilities of: (1) combining TKIs to broaden the spectrum of vascular growth factor receptor isoforms that are affected, and (2) targeting drug delivery to cancers when resistance is apparent. The impracticalities of conjoint TKI use include dosing cost, disparate commercial pharmaceutical sources, and a broadening of the side effect profile. Targeting of TKI delivery to permit local increases in drug dosing in the cancer microenvironment to offset

ABC transporter action, for example, is presently limited by the lack of availability of effective targeting moieties. Local delivery would also improve the side effect profile.

A third possibility that may improve anti-angiogenic properties of TKIs would be elimination of the proangiogenic contribution in treated patients of physiological concentrations of thyroid hormone, specifically, L-thyroxine (T_4). A practical formula for doing so, with maintenance of the euthyroid state, has been described [18]. As noted, certain TKIs may induce hypothyroidism [19–21]. Untreated, the latter may slow cancer growth, but undesirably leaves the affected patient in a hypometabolic state.

References

[1] Carlisle B, Demko N, Freeman G, Hakala A, MacKinnon N, Ramsay T, Hey S, London AJ, Kimmelman J. Benefit, risk, and outcomes in drug development: a systematic review of sunitinib. J Natl Cancer Inst 2016;108(1).

[2] Goodman VL, Rock EP, Dagher R, Ramchandani RP, Abraham S, Gobburu JV, Booth BP, Verbois SL, Morse DE, Liang CY, Chidambaram N, Jiang JX, Tang S, Mahjoob K, Justice R, Pazdur R. Approval summary: sunitinib for the treatment of imatinib refractory or intolerant gastrointestinal stromal tumors and advanced renal cell carcinoma. Clin Cancer Res 2007;13(5):1367–73.

[3] Escudier B, Eisen T, Stadler WM, Szczylik C, Oudard S, Staehler M, Negrier S, Chevreau C, Desai AA, Rolland F, Demkow T, Hutson TE, Gore M, Anderson S, Hofilena G, Shan M, Pena C, Lathia C, Bukowski RM. Sorafenib for treatment of renal cell carcinoma: Final efficacy and safety results of the phase III treatment approaches in renal cancer global evaluation trial. J Clin Oncol 2009;27(20):3312–8.

[4] Luidens MK, Mousa SA, Davis FB, Lin HY, Davis PJ. Thyroid hormone and angiogenesis. Vascul Pharmacol 2010;52(3–4):142–5.

[5] Mousa SA, Lin HY, Tang HY, Hercbergs A, Luidens MK, Davis PJ. Modulation of angiogenesis by thyroid hormone and hormone analogues: implications for cancer management. Angiogenesis 2014;17(3):463–9.

[6] Davis PJ, Davis FB, Mousa SA, Luidens MK, Lin HY. Membrane receptor for thyroid hormone: physiologic and pharmacologic implications. Annu Rev Pharmacol Toxicol 2011;51:99–115.

[7] Davis PJ, Goglia F, Leonard JL. Nongenomic actions of thyroid hormone. Nat Rev Endocrinol 2016;12(2):111–21.

 [8] Wells SA Jr, Gosnell JE, Gagel RF, Moley J, Pfister D, Sosa JA, Skinner M, Krebs A, Vasselli J, Schlumberger M. Vandetanib for the treatment of patients with locally advanced or metastatic hereditary medullary thyroid cancer. J Clin Oncol 2010;28(5):767–72.

 [9] Cabanillas ME, Hu MI, Jimenez C. Medullary thyroid cancer in the era of tyrosine kinase inhibitors: to treat or not to treat--and with which drug--those are the questions. J Clin Endocrinol Metab 2014;99(12):4390–6.

[10] Aslam S, Eisen T. Vascular endothelial growth factor receptor tyrosine kinase inhibitors in metastatic renal cell cancer: latest results and clinical implications. Ther Adv Med Oncol 2013;5(6):324–33.

[11] Noonan S, Man Wong K, Jimeno A. Nintedanib, a novel triple angiokinase inhibitor for the treatment of non-small cell lung cancer. Drugs Today (Barc) 2015;51(6):357–66.

[12] Wang Z, Wang M, Yang F, Nie W, Chen F, Xu J, Guan X. Multitargeted antiangiogenic tyrosine kinase inhibitors combined to chemotherapy in metastatic breast cancer: a systematic review and meta-analysis. Eur J Clin Pharmacol 2014;70(5):531–8.

[13] Shi L, Zhang S, Wu H, Zhang L, Dai X, Hu J, Xue J, Liu T, Liang Y, Wu G. MiR-200c increases the radiosensitivity of non-small-cell lung cancer cell line A549 by targeting VEGF-VEGFR2 pathway. PLoS One 2013;8(10):e78344.

[14] Iacovelli R, Massari F, Albiges L, Loriot Y, Massard C, Fizazi K, Escudier B. Evidence and clinical relevance of tumor flare in patients who discontinue tyrosine kinase inhibitors for treatment of metastatic renal cell carcinoma. Eur Urol 2015;68(1):154–60.

[15] Nurwidya F, Takahashi F, Murakami A, Kobayashi I, Kato M, Shukuya T, Tajima K, Shimada N, Takahashi K. Acquired resistance of non-small cell lung cancer to epidermal growth factor receptor tyrosine kinase inhibitors. Respir Investig 2014;52(2):82–91.

[16] Anreddy N, Gupta P, Kathawala RJ, Patel A, Wurpel JN, Chen ZS. Tyrosine kinase inhibitors as reversal agents for ABC transporter mediated drug resistance. Molecules 2014;19(9):13848–77.

[17] Bronte G, Bronte E, Novo G, Pernice G, Lo Vullo F, Musso E, Bronte F, Gulotta E, Rizzo S, Rolfo C, Silvestris N, Bazan V, Novo S, Russo A. Conquests and perspectives of cardio-oncology in the field of tumor angiogenesis-targeting tyrosine kinase inhibitor-based therapy. Expert Opin Drug Saf 2015;14(2):253–67.

[18] Hercbergs A, Johnson RE, Ashur-Fabian O, Garfield DH, Davis PJ. Medically induced euthyroid hypothyroxinemia may extend survival in compassionate need cancer patients: an observational study. Oncologist 2015;20(1):72–6.

[19] Bailey EB, Tantravahi SK, Poole A, Agarwal AM, Straubhar AM, Batten JA, Patel SB, Wells CE, Stenehjem DD, Agarwal N. Correlation of degree of hypothyroidism with survival outcomes in patients with metastatic renal cell carcinoma receiving vascular endothelial growth factor receptor tyrosine kinase inhibitors. Clin Genitourin Cancer 2015;13(3):e131–7.

[20] Riesenbeck LM, Bierer S, Hoffmeister I, Kopke T, Papavassilis P, Hertle L, Thielen B, Herrmann E. Hypothyroidism correlates with a better prognosis in metastatic renal cancer patients treated with sorafenib or sunitinib. World J Urol 2011;29(6):807–13.

[21] Schmidinger M, Vogl UM, Bojic M, Lamm W, Heinzl H, Haitel A, Clodi M, Kramer G, Zielinski CC. Hypothyroidism in patients with renal cell carcinoma: blessing or curse? Cancer 2011;117(3):534–44.

CHAPTER 9

Tetraiodothyroacetic Acid at Integrin αvβ3: A Model of Pharmaceutical Anti-Angiogenesis

Paul J. Davis and Shaker A. Mousa

Contents

INTRODUCTION

The proangiogenic properties of thyroid hormone (L-thyroxine, T_4; 3,5,3'-triiodo-L-thyronine, T_3) have been defined by a number of laboratories in the heart [1,2] or in model systems, such as the chick chorioallantoic membrane (CAM) [3] or wound–healing and tubule formation with human endothelial cells [4]. Studies of the proangiogenic properties of thyroid hormone in the CAM model were essential to the definition of the plasma membrane receptor for thyroid hormone on the extracellular domain of an integrin,

Anti-Angiogenesis Strategies in Cancer Therapies
http://dx.doi.org/10.1016/B978-0-12-802576-5.00009-7

αvβ3 [5]. This integrin is primarily expressed by rapidly dividing endothelial cells and by tumor cells [6]. The proangiogenic activity of the hormone, primarily of T_4 when effects of physiological concentrations of T_4 and T_3 were compared, is an example of a nongenomic hormonal action. Nongenomic actions are those that do not require a primary interaction of thyroid hormone with a well-defined nuclear thyroid hormone receptor (TR) [7]. Acting at this thyroid hormone receptor on integrin αvβ3, tetraiodothyroacetic acid (tetrac), the naturally occurring deaminated analog of T_4, was shown to block the binding of both T_4 and T_3 to the integrin [5] and to inhibit the proangiogenesis action of thyroid hormone in the CAM [3,5]. The vascular supply to a variety of human tumor xenografts was shown to be downregulated by tetrac [6,8,9], and this was initially interpreted by us to reflect only the interruption of the binding of thyroid hormone by αvβ3. However, in 2008 we found that in the *absence* of thyroid hormone, tetrac blocked the angiogenesis induced by vascular endothelial growth factor (VEGF) and by basic fibroblast growth factor (bFGF; FGF2) in the CAM and in an endothelial cell microtubule formation assay [10]. While these observations may simply have reflected interruption of cell surface protein crosstalk between the integrin and adjacent vascular growth factor receptors, they raised the possibility that tetrac had unique anti-angiogenic properties. We review here the evidence that this is the case.

Tetrac and its reformulation as a covalently linked targeting moiety on a nanoparticle are hormone-drugs that act at a single cellular target site that is linked intracellularly to the expression of multiple angiogenesis-relevant genes, to function of plasma membrane growth factor receptors and to a variety of other factors or mechanisms involved in blood vessel formation [11–13]. Unmodified tetrac is a low-grade thyromimetic when it achieves the intracellular space [14]. This contrasts with its actions at αvβ3 as a thyroid hormone antagonist. In order to restrict the activities of tetrac to the integrin, we reformulated the hormone analog as described earlier. The nanoparticle to which tetrac is chemically bonded is of sufficient size to reduce its internalization by

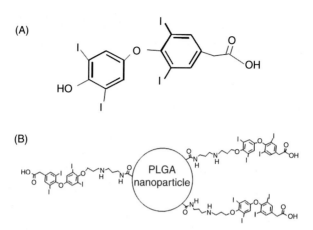

Figure 9.1 Chemical structures of unmodified tetraiodothyroacetic acid (tetrac) (A) and nanoparticulate tetrac (NDAT or Nanotetrac) (B). An ether bond involving the outer ring hydroxyl group joins tetrac to a linker molecule which, in turn, is attached by an imbedded amide bond to the nanoparticle. Multiple tetrac moieties are bonded to the surface of the PLGA, enabling access of tetrac to its receptor groove in the extracellular domain of integrin αvβ3.

cells [6,15]. Attached by an ether bond to a diaminopropane linker that is in turn bound to a 150–250 nm poly(lactide-co-glycolide) (PLGA) nanoparticle, tetrac as Nano-diamino-tetrac (also called NDAT, Nanotetrac, Fig. 9.1) acquired useful properties beyond those that accompany its restriction to the extracellular space [6,13]. Among these mechanistic assets were increased potency and integrin-initiated/dependent actions on a broader spectrum of differentially regulated genes, some of which were angiogenesis-relevant, such as epidermal growth factor receptor (*EGFR*).

Our analysis here of NDAT as an anti-angiogenic agent for use in the setting of cancer involves consideration of certain qualities that are ideal for, if not essential to, such pharmaceuticals. Among these qualities are anti-angiogenic actions by more than a single mechanism, high relevance to the molecular basis of tumor-relevant angiogenesis, low risk of intratumoral hemorrhage, and a favorable side effect profile. It is also desirable for idealized anti-angiogenic agents applicable to oncology that the emergence of drug resistance be limited.

THYROID HORMONE IS A PROANGIOGENIC AGENT AND TETRAC IS AN ANTI-ANGIOGENIC AGENT

In the CAM model, T_4 at physiological free hormone concentrations and T_3 at supraphysiologic concentrations increase vascularization by threefold within 72 h [3,5]. This threefold increase is similar to that obtained with FGF2. Covalently bound to agarose such that it is excluded from the intracellular space, T_4 reproduces the proangiogenic effect of unmodified thyroid hormone. Thus, the effect is initiated on the cell exterior. Tetrac inhibited the actions of unmodified thyroid hormone and of agarose-T_4 on angiogenesis, reflecting the blockade of T_4-binding sites on the cell surface. Pharmacologic inhibitors of mitogen-activated protein kinase (MAPK; ERK1/2) and of protein kinase C also blocked thyroid hormone-induced angiogenesis.

RT-PCR studies revealed that thyroid hormone stimulated *FGF2* gene expression within 6 h. Consequent measurement of medium FGF2 protein content confirmed cellular release of this angiogenic factor. Vascular sprouting [16] was thus a function of initiation at the plasma membrane of a nongenomic thyroid hormone effect that involved specific vascular growth factor gene transcription, translation, and release of the product. All of these steps were inhibited by tetrac.

Against this functional background, the existence of a cell surface receptor for thyroid hormone and tetrac relevant to angiogenesis was defined on the extracellular domain of integrin $\alpha v \beta 3$ [5]. GC-1 [17] and diiodothyropropionic acid (DITPA) [18] are other thyroid hormone analogs that were also shown to be proangiogenic. The blood vessel actions of these congeners was also blocked by tetrac.

Using the CAM, a mouse Matrigel plug assay and a human dermal microvascular endothelial cell (HDMEC) microtubule formation model, we examined the possibility that unmodified tetrac had anti-angiogenic activity in the absence of T_4 and T_3 [16]. The addition of VEGF or FGF2 to these models expectedly induced angiogenesis. Tetrac at up to 10 μM inhibited these actions of the vascular growth factor proteins by more than 50%. Interestingly, low concentrations of tetrac (1–3 μM) decreased the abundance of angiopoietin-2 (Ang-2) in the system but did not affect Ang-1. Ang-2 protein destabilizes vascular beds in anticipation of angiogenesis, whereas Ang-1 stabilizes existing vascular networking. The expression of several matrix metalloproteinase genes induced by VEGF that is consistent with preangiogenic destabilization of vascular beds was also inhibited by tetrac. The existence of this panel of anti-angiogenic actions of tetrac was consistent with its disruption of crosstalk between the integrin and the nearby VEGF receptors (VEGFRs) and FGFRs that has been described by others. Thus, in the absence of thyroid hormone, tetraiodothyroacetic acid demonstrated broadly based anti-angiogenic activity in a variety of models.

TETRAC, NDAT, AND ANGIOGENESIS-RELEVANT GENE EXPRESSION AND microRNA EXPRESSION

We have noted earlier that unmodified tetrac is internalized by cells and that within the cell, tetrac has low-grade T_4-like activity, and tetrac may be converted to triiodothyroacetic acid (triac), a thyroid hormone analog that is also thyromimetic [14,19]. Reformulation of tetrac as NDAT minimized cell uptake of the intact complex, and the resultant compound was restricted to the extracellular space and was found to have desirable additional biologic activities not previously obtained with tetrac.

In two human cancer cell lines, microarray studies revealed that both tetrac and NDAT inhibited expression of *VEGF-A* [20]; VEGF-A protein is a principal inducer of the porous blood vessels associated with cancers [21]. Tetrac and NDAT were found to increase transcription of thrombospondin 1 (*THBS1, TSP1*). TSP1 is a host protein that suppresses angiogenesis and is invariably suppressed in cancer cells. NDAT, but not tetrac, also decreased expression of *EGFR*, the gene product of which mediates actions of EGF on angiogenesis and has other functions critical to tumor cell biology. Acting at the integrin, NDAT, but not tetrac, downregulated expression of *NFκB* via the integrin and NFκB deactivation is recognized to be an anti-angiogenic target [22,23]. We know that thyroid hormone may also regulate transcription of the *αv* gene [24], but it is not yet clear at what cellular site this action is initiated, that is, plasma membrane αvβ3 versus nuclear TR.

In microRNA (miR) studies, NDAT has been shown to increase breast cancer cell content of miR-15A by 10-fold [25]. miR-15A is anti-angiogenic by a VEGF-dependent mechanism [26]. NDAT decreases miR-21 by 50% and miR-21 is a proangiogenic factor in certain tumor cells [27].

Mechanisms implicated in anti-angiogenic activity of NDAT are summarized in Table 9.1.

Table 9.1 Cellular/molecular mechanisms by which NDAT is anti-angiogenic

Angiogenesis-relevant target	Action
bFGF transcription	↓
VEGF-A transcription	↓
EGFR transcription	↓
TSP1 (*THBS1*) transcription	↑
miR-21 transcription	↓
miR-15A transcription	↑
Cellular bFGF abundance	↓
Cellular Ang-2 abundance	↓
Cellular MMP-9 abundance	↓
Integrin αvβ3—bFGFR crosstalk	↓
Integrin αvβ3—VEGFR crosstalk	↓
Integrin αvβ3—PDGFR crosstalk	↓
Cellular release of bFGF	↓
Endothelial cell motility in response to cue	↓
Proangiogenic activity of thyroid hormone	↓

Transcription measurements were made in breast cancer cells [33]. Crosstalk measurements were made in the CAM assay. See text for details of mechanisms involved in actions of NDAT reported in this table.

TETRAC, NDAT, AND ACTIONS OF VASCULAR GROWTH FACTORS

Inhibition of the actions of VEGF and bFGF [10] in preclinical models were the first anti-angiogenic effects of tetrac to be described, as noted earlier. We have also shown that the proangiogenic action of platelet-derived growth factor (PDGF) in a microtubule formation assay is blocked by tetrac (S.A. Mousa, unpublished observations). These actions at least in part appeared to involve crosstalk between the integrin and nearby growth factor-specific receptors on the cell surface.

Epidermal growth factor (EGF) is also involved in tumor-relevant angiogenesis, as has been shown in non-small cell lung carcinoma [28]. Interestingly, such actions of EGF may occur in conjunction with VEGFR [29]. We have shown that thyroid hormone may potentiate the activity of EGF at its receptor (EGFR) [30], and tetrac is an inhibitor of such activity. It is not yet clear whether such actions are specifically involved in blood vessel formation. It may be noted, however, that *c-fos* gene expression is a recognized downstream consequence of EGF action in tumor cells and c-fos is implicated in angiogenesis [31]. Signal transduction factors involved in EGF activity include MAPK and STAT3 [30,32] and the activity of these factors is downregulated by tetrac and NDAT. Transcription of the *EGFR* gene [33] is also downregulated by NDAT, but not by tetrac. Inhibition of EGF actions by tetrac formulations may involve changes in the functional capacity of EGFR and in the abundance of the EGFR protein.

TETRAC AND NDAT ACTIONS ON ENDOTHELIAL CELLS

Endothelial cell migration toward a vitronectin cue is stimulated by thyroid hormone [34], as shown in Boyden chamber studies. This action is blocked by NDAT and unmodified tetrac. Thus, this is an integrin αvβ3-mediated effect. The cell migration contribution is essential to the proangiogenic activity of thyroid hormone and to the anti-angiogenic effect of NDAT.

ANTI-ANGIOGENESIS OF NDAT IN THE RETINA

The anti-angiogenic effect of NDAT on retinal neovascularization has been studied in oxygen-induced retinopathy in the intact newborn mouse [35]. Administered by intravitreal or systemic routes, NDAT blocked new blood vessel formation. In this model of diabetic retinopathy, NDAT and tetrac in vitro were also shown to inhibit the proangiogenic activity of VEGF and erythropoietin [35].

ANTI-ANGIOGENESIS OF NDAT IN HUMAN TUMOR XENOGRAFTS

NDAT has anti-proliferative actions on a variety of cancer cell lines, as noted earlier. The hemoglobin content of xenografts of such cells is a parameter of vascularity/angiogenesis. Systemically administered NDAT has regularly resulted in a decrease of 50% or more in xenograft vascularity. The xenografts include those from cancer cell lines derived from human lung [36,37], pancreas [38], kidney [8], glioma/glioblastoma (T. Sudha, unpublished observations), and medullary thyroid carcinoma [20]. Recent histologic studies of glioblastoma xenografts exposed to systemic NDAT for 10 days have shown loss of 95% of blood vessel content (T. Sudha, unpublished observations). The devascularization is very systematic, in that there is no evidence of intratumoral hemorrhage. The loss of vascularity was associated with widespread tumor necrosis.

ACTION OF NDAT ON MECHANISMS OF VASCULAR SPROUTING

Thyroid hormone stimulates matrix metalloproteinase-9 (*MMP9*) gene expression [39]. MMPs, such as MMP-2 and MMP-9 are factors involved in preparing vascular beds for angiogenesis [40] and tetrac blocks the induction of *MMP9* expression by thyroid hormone [39]. We have noted earlier that Ang-2 elaboration—important to the destabilization of vascular beds in anticipation of sprouting—is decreased by tetrac.

PHARMACODYNAMICS OF NDAT

Anti-angiogenic activity of NDAT is optimized at 10^{-7}–10^{-6} M in the CAM model [6]. It is the actual tetrac concentration that is specified here, namely, about 8% of the mass of NDAT. Pharmacodynamics of NDAT as an anti-proliferative cancer chemotherapeutic agent have been studied in vitro in a cell culture perfusion bellows system [41]; in this model, the threshold tetrac (in NDAT) concentration is 10^{-9} M and maximal anti-proliferative activity against several human cancer cell lines is obtained at 10^{-7}–10^{-6} M. This is consistent with anti-angiogenesis studies in the CAM model.

The distribution of NDAT is throughout the extracellular space. The agent crosses the blood-brain barrier with at least 25% efficiency in mice bearing orthotopic glioma (M.A. Vogelbaum, unpublished observations). The PLGA nanoparticle is biodegradable in plasma. The chemical removal of lactate and glycolic acids from the PLGA nanoparticle linked to tetrac occurs in blood. The residue is tetrac linked to diaminopropane [15], a molecule with little bioactivity.

SIDE EFFECT PROFILE OF NDAT

NDAT has not caused hemorrhage in any human cancer xenografts that have been studied (S.A. Mousa, unpublished observations). The intact agent is excluded from the intracellular space. NDAT has caused no histopathologic changes in brain, heart, or kidneys of mice exposed for up to 2 weeks to high daily doses of the agent (S.A. Mousa, unpublished observations).

Angiogenesis is desirable at the sites of self-limited inflammation, for example, infection, or at wound-healing sites. Proangiogenic events at such sites may be inhibited by NDAT. These settings have not been studied preclinically, but we anticipate that the use of the agent in these settings will be contraindicated. The use of the agent in pregnancy will be contraindicated. Transplacental passage of NDAT has not been studied experimentally.

CONCLUSIONS

A large panel of intracellular and extracellular functions of cells is regulated by integrin $\alpha v\beta 3$. The transmembrane structural protein is differentially expressed/activated in dividing blood vessel cells and tumor cells, making the agent a candidate for targeting angiogenesis in oncology. Recognition of thyroid hormone-tetrac receptor site on $\alpha v\beta 3$ [5,6] brought with it a recognition of control from the integrin of expression of differentially regulated, angiogenesis-relevant genes, as well as modulation of function of adjacent vascular growth factor receptors. Previously, these functions of the integrin were not fully appreciated.

NDAT is a model of an anti-angiogenic agent focused on a single, specific small molecule receptor site on the extracellular domain of a cell surface protein, but has extensive downstream and plasma membrane actions that are relevant to new blood vessel formation. From this single site, NDAT opposes effects of VEGF, FGF2 and PDGF at their plasma membrane receptors, inhibits expression of genes for *VEGF-A* and *EGFR*, upregulates transcription of *TSP1*, and selectively regulates miRNAs that control angiogenesis, and decreases endothelial cell motility.

REFERENCES

[1] Tomanek RJ, Doty MK, Sandra A. Early coronary angiogenesis in response to thyroxine: growth characteristics and upregulation of basic fibroblast growth factor. Circ Res 1998;82(5):587–93.

[2] Chen JH, Ortmeier SB, Savinova OV, Nareddy VB, Beyer AJ, Wang DJ, Gerdes AM. Thyroid hormone induces sprouting angiogenesis in adult heart of hypothyroid mice through the PDGF-Akt pathway. J Cell Mol Med 2012;16(11):2726–35.

[3] Davis FB, Mousa SA, O'Connor L, Mohamed S, Lin HY, Cao HJ, Davis PJ. Proangiogenic action of thyroid hormone is fibroblast growth factor-dependent and is initiated at the cell surface. Circ Res 2004;94(11):1500–6.

[4] Liu X, Zheng N, Shi YN, Yuan J, Li L. Thyroid hormone induced angiogenesis through the integrin $\alpha v\beta 3$/protein kinase D/histone deacetylase 5 signaling pathway. J Mol Endocrinol 2014;52(3):245–54.

[5] Bergh JJ, Lin HY, Lansing L, Mohamed SN, Davis FB, Mousa S, Davis PJ. Integrin $\alpha v\beta 3$ contains a cell surface receptor site for thyroid hormone

that is linked to activation of mitogen-activated protein kinase and induction of angiogenesis. Endocrinology 2005;146(7):2864–71.

[6] Davis PJ, Davis FB, Mousa SA, Luidens MK, Lin HY. Membrane receptor for thyroid hormone: physiologic and pharmacologic implications. Annu Rev Pharmacol Toxicol 2011;51:99–115.

[7] Cheng SY, Leonard JL, Davis PJ. Molecular aspects of thyroid hormone actions. Endocr Rev 2010;31(2):139–70.

[8] Yalcin M, Bharali DJ, Lansing L, Dyskin E, Mousa SS, Hercbergs A, Davis FB, Davis PJ, Mousa SA. Tetraidothyroacetic acid (tetrac) and tetrac nanoparticles inhibit growth of human renal cell carcinoma xenografts. Anticancer Res 2009;29(10):3825–31.

[9] Yalcin M, Bharali DJ, Dyskin E, Dier E, Lansing L, Mousa SS, Davis FB, Davis PJ, Mousa SA. Tetraiodothyroacetic acid and tetraiodothyroacetic acid nanoparticle effectively inhibit the growth of human follicular thyroid cell carcinoma. Thyroid 2010;20(3):281–6.

[10] Mousa SA, Bergh JJ, Dier E, Rebbaa A, O'Connor LJ, Yalcin M, Aljada A, Dyskin E, Davis FB, Lin HY, Davis PJ. Tetraiodothyroacetic acid, a small molecule integrin ligand, blocks angiogenesis induced by vascular endothelial growth factor and basic fibroblast growth factor. Angiogenesis 2008;11(2):183–90.

[11] Rajabi M, Srinivasan M, Mousa SA. Nanobiomaterials in drug delivery. In: Grumezescu A, editor. Nanobiomaterials in drug delivery: applications of nanobiomaterials, vol. 9. Amsterdam: Elsevier; 2016. p. 1–39.

[12] Srinivasan M, Rajabi M, Mousa SA. Multifunctional nanomaterials and their applications in drug delivery and cancer therapy. Nanomaterials 2015;5(4):1690–703.

[13] Srinivasan M, Rajabi M, Mousa SA. Nanobiomaterials in cancer therapy. In: Grumezescu A, editor. Nanobiomaterials in cancer therapy: applications of nanobiomaterials, vol. 7. Amsterdam: Elsevier; 2016. p. 57–89.

[14] Moreno M, de Lange P, Lombardi A, Silvestri E, Lanni A, Goglia F. Metabolic effects of thyroid hormone derivatives. Thyroid 2008;18(2): 239–53.

[15] Bharali DJ, Yalcin M, Davis PJ, Mousa SA. Tetraiodothyroacetic acid-conjugated PLGA nanoparticles: a nanomedicine approach to treat drug-resistant breast cancer. Nanomedicine (Lond) 2013;8(12):1943–54.

[16] Mousa SA, Davis FB, Mohamed S, Davis PJ, Feng X. Pro-angiogenesis action of thyroid hormone and analogs in a three-dimensional in vitro microvascular endothelial sprouting model. Int Angiol 2006;25(4): 407–13.

[17] Mousa SA, O'Connor LJ, Bergh JJ, Davis FB, Scanlan TS, Davis PJ. The proangiogenic action of thyroid hormone analogue GC-1 is initiated at an integrin. J Cardiovasc Pharmacol 2005;46(3):356–60.

[18] Mousa SA, O'Connor L, Davis FB, Davis PJ. Proangiogenesis action of the thyroid hormone analog 3,5-diiodothyropropionic acid (DITPA) is initiated at the cell surface and is integrin mediated. Endocrinology 2006;147(4):1602–7.

[19] Agrawal NK, Goyal R, Rastogi A, Naik D, Singh SK. Thyroid hormone resistance. Postgrad Med J 2008;84(995):473–7.

[20] Yalcin M, Dyskin E, Lansing L, Bharali DJ, Mousa SS, Bridoux A, Hercbergs AH, Lin HY, Davis FB, Glinsky GV, Glinskii A, Ma J, Davis PJ, Mousa SA. Tetraiodothyroacetic acid (tetrac) and nanoparticulate tetrac arrest growth of medullary carcinoma of the thyroid. J Clin Endocrinol Metab 2010;95(4):1972–80.

[21] Nagy JA, Dvorak AM, Dvorak HF. Vascular hyperpermeability, angiogenesis, and stroma generation. Cold Spring Harb Perspect Med 2012;2(2):a006544.

[22] Palenski TL, Gurel Z, Sorenson CM, Hankenson KD, Sheibani N. Cyp1B1 expression promotes angiogenesis by suppressing NF-κB activity. Am J Physiol Cell Physiol 2013;305(11):C1170–84.

[23] Omar HA, Arafa El-SA, Salama SA, Arab HH, Wu CH, Weng JR. OSU-A9 inhibits angiogenesis in human umbilical vein endothelial cells via disrupting Akt-NF-κB and MAPK signaling pathways. Toxicol Appl Pharmacol 2013;272(3):616–24.

[24] Pathak A, Sinha RA, Mohan V, Mitra K, Godbole MM. Maternal thyroid hormone before the onset of fetal thyroid function regulates reelin and downstream signaling cascade affecting neocortical neuronal migration. Cerebral Cortex 2011;21(1):11–21.

[25] Mousa SA, Thangirala S, Lin HY, Tang HY, Glinsky GV, Davis PJ. MicroRNA-21 and microRNA-15A expression in human breast cancer (MDA-MB-231) cells exposed to nanoparticulate tetraiodothyroacetic acid (Nanotetrac). ENDO Annual Meeting; June 21–24, 2014; Chicago.

[26] Sun CY, She XM, Qin Y, Chu ZB, Chen L, Ai LS, Zhang L, Hu Y. MiR-15a and miR-16 affect the angiogenesis of multiple myeloma by targeting VEGF. Carcinogenesis 2013;34(2):426–35.

[27] Zhao DL, Tu YF, Wan L, Bu LH, Huang T, Sun XL, Wang K, Shen BZ. In vivo monitoring of angiogenesis inhibition via down-regulation of miR-21 in a VEGFR2-luc murine breast cancer model using bioluminescent imaging. Plos One 2013;8(8):e71472.

[28] de Mello RA, Madureira P, Carvalho LS, Araujo A, O'Brien M, Popat S. EGFR and KRAS mutations, and ALK fusions: current developments and personalized therapies for patients with advanced non-small-cell lung cancer. Pharmacogenomics 2013;14(14):1765–77.

[29] Bruce D, Tan PH. Vascular endothelial growth factor receptors and the therapeutic targeting of angiogenesis in cancer: where do we go from here? Cell Commun Adhes 2011;18(5):85–103.

[30] Shih A, Zhang SL, Cao HJ, Tang HY, Davis FB, Davis PJ, Lin HY. Disparate effects of thyroid hormone on actions of epidermal growth factor and transforming growth factor-alpha are mediated by 3',5'-cyclic adenosine 5'-monophosphate-dependent protein kinase II. Endocrinology 2004;145(4):1708–17.

[31] Li YQ, Tao KS, Ren N, Wang YH. Effect of *c-fos* antisense probe on prostaglandin E2-induced upregulation of vascular endothelial growth factor mRNA in human liver cancer cells. World J Gastroenterol 2005;11(28):4427–30.

[32] Lin HY, Shih A, Davis FB, Davis PJ. Thyroid hormone promotes the phosphorylation of STAT3 and potentiates the action of epidermal growth factor in cultured cells. Biochem J 1999;338(Pt 2):427–32.

[33] Glinskii AB, Glinsky GV, Lin HY, Tang HY, Sun M, Davis FB, Luidens MK, Mousa SA, Hercbergs AH, Davis PJ. Modification of survival pathway gene expression in human breast cancer cells by tetraiodothyroacetic acid (tetrac). Cell Cycle 2009;8(21):3562–70.

[34] Mousa SA, Lin HY, Tang HY, Hercbergs A, Luidens MK, Davis PJ. Modulation of angiogenesis by thyroid hormone and hormone analogues: implications for cancer management. Angiogenesis 2014;17(3):463–9.

[35] Yoshida T, Gong J, Xu Z, Wei Y, Duh EJ. Inhibition of pathological retinal angiogenesis by the integrin αvβ3 antagonist tetraiodothyroacetic acid (tetrac). Exp Eye Res 2012;94(1):41–8.

[36] Mousa SA, Yalcin M, Bharali DJ, Meng R, Tang HY, Lin HY, Davis FB, Davis PJ. Tetraiodothyroacetic acid and its nanoformulation inhibit thyroid hormone stimulation of non-small cell lung cancer cells in vitro and its growth in xenografts. Lung Cancer 2012;76(1):39–45.

[37] Meng R, Tang HY, Westfall J, London D, Cao JH, Mousa SA, Luidens M, Hercbergs A, Davis FB, Davis PJ, Lin HY. Crosstalk between integrin αvβ3 and estrogen receptor-α is involved in thyroid hormone–induced proliferation in human lung carcinoma cells. PLoS One 2011;6(11):e27547.

[38] Yalcin M, Lin HY, Sudha T, Bharali DJ, Meng R, Tang HY, Davis FB, Stain SC, Davis PJ, Mousa SA. Response of human pancreatic cancer cell xenografts to tetraiodothyroacetic acid nanoparticles. Horm Cancer 2013;4(3):176–85.

[39] Cohen K, Flint N, Shalev S, Erez D, Baharal T, Davis PJ, Hercbergs A, Ellis M, Ashur-Fabian O. Thyroid hormone regulates adhesion, migration and matrix metalloproteinase 9 activity via αvβ3 integrin in myeloma cells. Oncotarget 2014;5(15):6312–22.

[40] Chen Q, Jin M, Yang F, Zhu J, Xiao Q, Zhang L. Matrix metalloproteinases: inflammatory regulators of cell behaviors in vascular formation and remodeling. Mediators Inflamm 2013;2013:928315.

[41] Lin HY, Landersdorfer CB, London D, Meng R, Lim CU, Lin C, Lin S, Tang HY, Brown D, Van Scoy B, Kulawy R, Queimado L, Drusano GL, Louie A, Davis FB, Mousa SA, Davis PJ. Pharmacodynamic modeling of anti-cancer activity of tetraiodothyroacetic acid in a perfused cell culture system. PLoS Comput Biol 2011;7(2):e1001073.

CHAPTER 10

Anti-Angiogenesis Therapy and its Combination with Chemotherapy: Impact on Primary Tumor and its Metastasis

Shaker A. Mousa, Thangirala Sudha and Paul J. Davis

Contents

INTRODUCTION

Angiogenesis is an inherent body process that is stimulated by tissue demands for oxygen and for nutrients. The process is carefully orchestrated by actions of host proangiogenic and anti-angiogenic factors. The nutritional and oxygenation needs of cancers that are less than 1 mm in diameter are met through the process of diffusion [1]. Additional growth requires tumor–relevant blood vessel

Anti-Angiogenesis Strategies in Cancer Therapies
http://dx.doi.org/10.1016/B978-0-12-802576-5.00010-3

formation. Thus, angiogenesis is a principal contributor to tumor growth and to metastasis.

A variety of anti-angiogenic treatments have evolved for use in conjunction with cytotoxic cancer chemotherapy. It would appear obvious that the addition of anti-angiogenic therapy would improve outcomes of chemotherapy-managed cancer patients, yet results of the recent AVADO [2] and RiBBON-1 [3] trials failed to disclose benefit of anti-angiogenic therapies to survival. The mechanisms of such failures can be understood at least in part by improved understanding of cancer-related blood vessel formation and maintenance in both primary and metastatic lesions.

In this chapter, the role of anti-angiogenic treatment in cancer as an adjunct to chemotherapy will be reviewed.

BIOMARKERS OF ANGIOGENESIS

Biomarkers are molecules or genes that can be practically monitored to track certain physiological or pathophysiological changes that occur in the body, including cancer. Biomarkers are an index of change, but usually, as well, they are participants in the process of interest. Anti-angiogenic therapies must affect a sufficient quantity or array of these biomarkers in order to diminish or arrest the progress of angiogenesis. The contribution of certain anti-angiogenic modalities to standard anti-cancer therapy must be also considered in the context of cost-benefit analysis. Monitoring of biomarkers may provide insight into this analysis in the course of preclinical and clinical trials of combinations of anti-angiogenic and standard chemotherapeutic drugs. A brief discussion of certain relevant biomarkers is provided here.

1. *Hypoxia inducible factor-1α:* Angiogenesis is initiated by a decline in oxygen supply to and oxygen tension (hypoxia) in the newly formed tumor. Hypoxia occurs as metabolic demand for supportive O_2 increases with cancer cell multiplication. Hypoxia leads to the tumor cell release of hypoxia inducible factor-1α (HIF-1α). The activity of HIF-1α promotes the progression of angiogenesis and metastases through induction of the release

of growth factors, such as vascular endothelial growth factor (VEGF), epidermal growth factor (EGF), and insulin-like growth factor-2 (IGF-2). Increased levels of HIF-1α and VEGF have been linked to increased mortality in cancer [4–6].

2. *Vascular endothelial growth factor*: VEGF, also known as vascular permeability factor, is responsible for the activation of the VEGF receptor (VEGFR) located on the surface of vascular endothelial cells. The VEGF family consists of VEGF-A, VEGF-B, VEGF-C, VEGF-D, and placental growth factor (PIGF). There are three types of VEGF tyrosine kinase receptors on the surface of endothelial cells, VEGFR-1, VEGFR-2, and VEGFR-3. Once VEGF ligand binds to its receptor, a series of intracellular signals is set off to initiate angiogenesis, endothelial cell migration, and permeability. VEGF-A binds to both VEGFRs-1 and -2, whereas VEGF-B and PIGF bind only to VEGFR-1. Once VEGF binds to its receptor, the activated VEGF receptor will stimulate the AKT/mTOR signaling pathway through phosphoinositide 3-kinase (PI3-K), leading to additional phosphorylation downstream and to the formation of mTOR (mammalian target of rapamycin) complexes [7,8]. This signaling pathway has complex proangiogenic effects, including stimulation of production of nitric oxide, angiopoietins and HIF-1α. Activated by VEGF, this pathway may also induce further VEGF production.

3. *Matrix metalloproteinases*: Matrix metalloproteinases (MMPs) are a group of enzymes that degrade the extracellular environment to facilitate new vessel formation, by allowing endothelial cell migration to and around the tissue surrounding the tumor [9].

IMPACT OF ANGIOGENESIS ON TUMOR GROWTH AND METASTASIS

The circulatory system is the primary route of spread of cancers to distant organs. Lymphatic vessels provide a pathway to local lymph nodes, after which cancer cells often travel through the blood. The extent of hematogenous versus lymphatic spread appears to depend on the origin and location of the primary tumor.

For example, bone and soft tissue tumors spread primarily through the blood, while melanoma, lung, and gastrointestinal tumors usually spread through the lymphatic system. In order for tumor cells to gain access to lymphatic or blood vessels, tumors need to promote angiogenesis and lymphangiogenesis into and around the tumor. Angiogenesis inhibitors are known to halt tumor growth and suppress tumor metastasis [10].

CURRENT ANTI-ANGIOGENIC THERAPIES

Angiogenesis is currently targeted with biologic agents and small molecules. The FDA has approved agents such as bevacizumab and sorafenib for use with chemotherapy in certain cancers. These anti-angiogenic interventions are approved only as adjuncts to chemotherapy and are not to be used alone to treat cancer. Due to the large variation in biomarkers involved in the angiogenesis process, many anti-angiogenic therapies vary by the types of factor(s) that they target. The major targets of current therapy are VEGF and vascular growth factor receptors. Other biomarkers such as HIF-1α and MMPs are major contributors to the angiogenic process, but are yet to be included as targets in current therapy. A brief discussion of relevant anti-angiogenic therapies is given subsequently.

Bevacizumab in Breast Cancer

In the E2100 trial published in 2007, paclitaxel versus paclitaxel plus bevacizumab for the treatment of metastatic breast cancer showed a significant increase in progression-free survival in the paclitaxel plus bevacizumab group (11.8 months) versus the paclitaxel group (5.9 months) [11]. Accelerated FDA approval of bevacizumab for metastatic breast cancer in 2008 was based on the results of the E2100 trial. The FDA requested that further trials be conducted to demonstrate that the addition of bevacizumab to chemotherapy provided an improvement in overall survival. The AVADO three-arm trial published in 2010 compared two doses of bevacizumab plus docetaxel versus placebo plus docetaxel for the first line treatment of HER-2 negative metastatic breast cancer. Results of the trial showed a significant increase in progression-free survival for the higher dose bevacizumab-treated group, but the overall survival analysis revealed little difference among the three groups [2]. The subsequent RiBBON trials in 2011 confirmed a lack of improvement in overall survival with the addition of bevacizumab to standard chemotherapy [3]. Based on the results of the AVADO and RiBBON trials, the FDA acted in late 2011 to remove the indication for bevacizumab in metastatic breast cancer [12].

Monoclonal Antibodies in Other Cancers

Currently, bevacizumab is FDA-approved for: (1) first-line treatment of metastatic non-small cell lung cancer in combination with carboplatin and paclitaxel; (2) first- and second-line treatment of metastatic colorectal cancer in combination with intravenous 5-fluorouracil-based chemotherapy; (3) metastatic renal cell carcinoma in combination with interferon-α; and (4) as a single agent in the treatment of adult glioblastoma with progressive disease in postchemotherapy patients.

VEGF-trap (aflibercept) is a recombinant fusion protein that binds VEGF-A and PlGF [13], inhibiting their binding to and activation of VEGF receptors. Aflibercept is currently FDA-approved for the treatment of patients with neovascular age-related macular degeneration [14]. In terms of its use in cancer, aflibercept has shown intermediate results and even poor results in the treatment of non-small cell lung cancer and pancreatic cancer. Lack of an FDA approval for cancer does not limit its potential use as an anti-angiogenic treatment for tumors. Aflibercept versus placebo has shown promising patient improvement in overall patient survival in an ongoing trial of the drug in combination with irinotecan and 5-fluorouracil in metastatic colorectal cancer after failure of an oxaliplatin based regimen (VELOUR) [15]. The agent has shown positive results in its adjunctive use in metastatic colon cancer patients in FDA Phase III trials.

AMG 386 is a peptide-Fc fusion protein that prevents the binding of angiopoietin-1 and angiopoietin-2 to Tie2 receptors [16]. This agent is showing potential for use in combination with chemotherapy for the treatment of ovarian cancer. AMG 386 is undergoing a Phase III clinical trial named Trinova-3: a study of AMG 386 or AMG 386 placebo in combination with paclitaxel and carboplatin to treat ovarian cancer [17]. Long term experience with the agent is not yet available.

Ramucirumab is a 100% humanized monoclonal antibody directed at VEGFR-2 and it prevents the binding of VEGF to this receptor. This agent showed anti-tumor and anti-angiogenic activity during FDA Phase I and II trials conducted on renal cell carcinoma, hepatocellular carcinoma, non-small cell lung cancer, and melanoma [18]. This agent differs from bevacizumab in that it targets a receptor that binds more than one growth factor isoform, whereas bevacizumab is directed at one vascular growth factor, preventing binding of the latter to VEGF receptors, such as VEGFR-2. Additional experience with the agent revealed failure to achieve primary endpoints in Phase III studies of women with metastatic breast cancer [19] and hepatic cancer [20].

DI17E6 is a monoclonal antibody to human αv integrin. Integrins are structural proteins of the plasma membrane that are primarily expressed by cancer cells and dividing blood vessel cells. The drug, itself, effectively reduced angiogenesis in prostate cancer by preventing cell adhesion and migration. DI17E6 was then used as a targeting agent for delivery of standard chemotherapy. In a preclinical study by Wagner and coworkers, DI17E6 was bonded to a doxorubicin-containing albumin nanoparticle. Compared with conventional drug delivery, the DI17E6-linked cytotoxic nanoparticle achieved an increased level of tumor chemotherapeutic agent [21].

There are numerous monoclonal antibodies in early Phase II anti-cancer trials, two of which, MetMAb and Pegdinetanib, have shown efficacy in preventing angiogenesis in non-small cell lung cancer and glioblastoma, respectively.

Tyrosine Kinase Inhibitors

Sunitinib (Sutent), a multireceptor tyrosine kinase inhibitor (TKI), is a small molecule that binds to and inhibits activation of receptors platelet derived growth factor receptor α (PDGFRα), PDGFRβ, VEGFR-1,VEGFR-2,VEGFR-3, stem cell factor receptor (KIT), Fms-like tyrosine kinase-3 (FLT-3), colony stimulating factor receptor type 1 (CSF-1R), and glial cell line derived neurotrophic factor receptor (RET). There is FDA approval for use of sunitinib in the treatment of gastrointestinal stromal tumors, renal cell carcinoma, and advanced pancreatic neuroendocrine tumors. Unlike biologic agents that require intravenous administration, sunitinib is administered orally [22,23].

Sorafenib (Nexavar) is a multireceptor TKI that is FDA-approved for treatment of nonresectable hepatocellular carcinoma [24] and advanced renal cell carcinoma. Among the cell surface targets of this agent are VEGFR-1, VEGFR-2, VEGFR-3, and PDGFRβ, KIT, FLT-3, and RET [25]. In a study by Escudier and coworkers that compared sorafenib to placebo in previously treated renal cell carcinoma patients, overall survival was not found to be statistically significantly improved [26].

Vandetanib (Caprelsa) is a TKI that binds to the EGF receptor, VEGF receptors, RET, protein tyrosine kinase 6, Tie2, EPH receptor kinases, and Src tyrosine kinases. Results of vandetanib action are a decrease in endothelial cell migration, proliferation, and survival, and, thereby, reduced neovascularization. Vandetanib is currently FDA-approved for the treatment of symptomatic or progressive medullary thyroid cancer in patients who have non-resectable, locally advanced or metastatic disease [27]. In a Phase II open label study of 30 patients with medullary carcinoma of the thyroid, vandetanib treatment achieved a partial anti-tumor response in 20% of patients and stabilized disease for 53% of patients at ≥ 24 weeks [28].

Pazopanib (Votrient) is a multi-TKI of VEGFR-1, VEGFR-2, VEGFR-3, PDGFRα, PDGFRβ, fibroblast growth factor receptor-1 (FGFR-1), FGFR-3, KIT, IL-2, and c-FMS [29]. Pazopanib is

FDA-approved for the management of renal cell carcinoma, based on the results of a Phase III trial comparing pazopanib versus placebo in adult patients with measurable, locally advanced, and/or metastatic renal cell carcinoma. The 435 patient trial involved randomization of patients into pazopanib or placebo groups and they were treated until endpoints of disease progression, toxicity, death, or patient withdrawal. Progression-free survival was significantly prolonged in the pazopanib-treated cohort (9.2 months, treated, vs. 4.2 months, placebo [30,31]).

Newer small molecule anti-angiogenic therapies that are in clinical trials include tivozanib (a VEGF receptor inhibitor), axitinib (a multi-kinase inhibitor), motesanib (a multi-kinase inhibitor), intedanib (a VEGFR-2/PDGFR/FGFR inhibitor), and brivanib (a VEGFR-2/FGFR-1 inhibitor).

PROBLEMS ENCOUNTERED WITH ANTI-ANGIOGENIC THERAPY

Currently FDA-approved anti-angiogenic therapies demonstrate some effectiveness in halting angiogenesis, but clearly fail to arrest it completely. Tumor metastasis and mortality continue to be observed with bevacizumab, sorafenib, and sunitinib treatments.

VEGF inhibition alone is insufficient to stop neovascularization. The multireceptor tyrosine kinases such as sunitinib and pazopanib slow angiogenesis, but fail to prevent the metastatic process. In addition, TKIs have important side effects in normal tissues and organs that at least in part reflect lack of specificity of action for tumor cells and cancer-relevant angiogenesis. Thus, anti-angiogenesis agents are needed that are specifically directed at multiple targets in the cancer-related process of angiogenesis.

DISTINCTIVE FEATURES OF TUMOR-RELATED ANGIOGENESIS
Blood Vessel Porosity

The leakiness of the vasculature serving cancers and its utility have been extensively demonstrated by Dvorak [32] and others. The provisionally porous nature of this vascularization is essential to early stroma formation that facilitates cancer cell migration, connective tissue formation, and ultimately, a mature vascularized stroma that provides long-term tumor support of established tumor. VEGF-A is a principal stimulator of the formation of this genre of porous blood vessels.

Razoxane and dexrazoxane are another set of agents with anti-angiogenic properties. They are thought to reduce the very permeable vessels within tumors and to reduce interstitial pressure surrounding the tumor site. In a study conducted to determine the anti-angiogenic effects of dexrazoxane, it was found that the agent causes an upregulation of THBS1 an endogenous inhibitor of neovascularization [33].

Interstitial Pressure Increase

As a tumor progresses, interstitial fluid pressure surrounding the tumor increases due to the increased permeability of vessels and the lack of lymphatic drainage. This increase in interstitial pressure is associated with hypoxia, which stimulates production of proangiogenic factors at the outer rim of the tumor where the transient increase in vessel permeability is most notable.

Angiogenesis and Thrombosis

Platelet activation and loose fibrin stroma formation are additional mechanisms by which tumor cells promote angiogenesis and metastasis, forming a coating of tumor cells. This process promotes tumor cell conjunction into small thrombi that can lodge in the vasculature [34]. Local protease activation and the coagulation system generate conditions or factors that support angiogenesis and tumor cell proliferation. It has been noted that heparin is effective in inhibiting the proliferation of endothelial cells and hindering angiogenesis via structural changes to fibrin networks surrounding tumors [35]. Low molecular weight heparin (LMWH) has been shown to be superior to unfractionated heparin (UFH) for this purpose. In a study comparing the two anti-coagulants, it was found that UFH enhanced the fibrin matrix and had a proangiogenic outcome whereas LMWH had an anti–angiogenic effect on the tumor [35]. It may be advantageous to add thrombosis prophylaxis to clinical anti–angiogenic therapy because of an increased risk of thromboembolism and clot formation that accompanies adminis-tration of anti–angiogenesis agents [36].

NOVEL ANTI-ANGIOGENESIS STRATEGIES

Angiogenesis that supports cancer has been treated with agents that inhibit one or a few of the many ways that tumors initiate an-giogenesis and progressively become metastatic. The revocation by the FDA of the treatment indication for bevacizumab in metastatic breast cancer is an example of failure of an agent with a narrow treatment goal. The need for therapies that target multiple recep-tors and biomarkers is a trend that has been producing a number of new agents that are showing promising results in clinical trials.

Tetrac, a derivative of thyroid hormone (L–thyroxine, T_4), and tet-rac reformulated as nanoparticles (Nanotetrac, Nano–diamino–tetrac, NDAT) have both shown anti–proliferative and anti–angiogenic action against cancer cells in preclinical studies. T_4 and T_3 (3,5,3′–triiodo-L–thyronine), the active form of thyroid hormone in the cell nu-cleus, are both capable of binding to a thyroid hormone receptor located on the extracellular domain of plasma membrane integrin $\alpha v \beta 3$. At this receptor, T_4 and T_3 are proangiogenic [37]. Tetrac and Nanotetrac have been tested in human lung cancer cells in vitro and in xenografts. Tetrac and Nanotetrac inhibited the binding of T_4 and T_3 to the hormone receptor on the integrin, blocked the proliferative effects of thyroid hormone on these tumor cells and, in xenografts, inhibited angiogenesis. Nanotetrac proved to be su-perior to unmodified tetrac in that it had broader effects on ma-lignant cell gene expression and was more potent [38–40]. Further studies with tetrac and Nanotetrac are needed to determine their longer term effects in xenografts.

Thalidomide (Thalomid), an anti–inflammatory, anti-angiogenic, and immunomodulatory agent, has been used to treat conditions such as cutaneous manifestations of erythema nodosum leprosum and, in combination with dexamethasone, to treat newly diagnosed multiple myeloma. This agent reduces the levels of tumor necrosis factor-α (TNF-α), increases the number of natural killer cells, increases interleukin-2 (IL-2), and decreases the proliferation of endothelial cells [41]. Thalidomide reduces angiogenesis by decreasing the secretion of proangiogenic factors such as VEGF and IL-6 into the tumor microenvironment. Thalidomide has been tested against both hematological malignancies and solid tumors, but the success found in thalidomide treatment of multiple myeloma has not been reproduced in hepatocellular and colorectal cancer solid tumors [42,43].

Lenalidomide (Revlimid) is another immunomodulatory drug that is used in the treatment of patients with refractory multiple myeloma—where lenalidomide is combined with dexamethasone—and for the treatment of myelodysplasia [44]. In a study comparing lenalidomide and dexamethasone versus placebo and dexamethasone for the treatment of relapsed multiple myeloma, complete or partial responses were observed in 61% of the lenalidomide group and 19.9% of the dexamethasone-only group [45].

The idea of linking chemotherapy agents with anti-VEGF receptor antibodies has also been employed and tested, with promising results. Wicki and coworkers used a VEGFR-2 antibody with doxorubicin to inhibit three tumor models in the intact mouse. It was found that the doxorubicin-linked VEGFR antibody provided better selectivity and suppression of the tumor vasculature than doxorubicin or VEGFR antibody alone [46]. The practice of using a highly expressed receptor on the surface of tumor cells to deliver chemotherapy allows for greater binding specificity and decreases the effects of chemotherapy-related adverse effects.

ANTI-ANGIOGENESIS AND NANOTARGETING

Conventional anti-angiogenic therapy has several limitations including emergence of drug resistance and side effects in uninvolved tissues that can create problems for a successful therapeutic strategy [47,48]. Recently, several nanoparticulate drugs have been developed that show anti-angiogenic properties [49,50]. These nanomedicines could be useful as an alternative strategy for the treatment of various cancers using anti-angiogenic therapy to suppress tumor angiogenesis [51,52]. Nanoparticles conjugated with a relevant targeting agent can direct anti-angiogenic agents to receptors for VEGF, for FGF and its receptors and to specific functions of MMPs, and tubulin. These targeted drug delivery systems allow them to deliver both anti-angiogenic molecules and anti-cancer drugs, facilitate drug penetration into extravascular tumor tissue and consequently increase drug efficacy and reduce the systemic toxicity [39,53]. Silica nanoparticles have been used as anti-angiogenic agents or as siRNA delivery vehicles for cancer therapy [54]. Chitosan nanoparticles have demonstrated their effectiveness in human hepatocellular carcinoma xenografts through anti-angiogenic mechanism involving VEGF and VEGFR-2 [55]. We have demonstrated potent anti-angiogenesis and effective tumor targeting with PLGA-diaminopropane-tetrac nanoparticles (Nanotetrac, Nano-diamino-tetrac, NDAT) and other strategies [56–59].

CONCLUSIONS

The future of oncology is shifting toward a multicomponent treatment approach involving both cytotoxic and noncytotoxic therapies. Conventional chemotherapeutic agents may eventually be administered more efficiently through the use of nanotechnology and targeted antibodies or targeting small molecules that recognize receptors on the surfaces of tumor cells or endothelial cells. Such modifications of standard chemotherapy administration will not only reduce the risk of systemic effects but also provide better survival outcomes for the cancer patient.

REFERENCES

[1] Singhal S, Vachani A, Antin-Ozerkis D, Kaiser LR, Albelda SM. Prognostic implications of cell cycle, apoptosis, and angiogenesis biomarkers in non-small cell lung cancer: a review. Clin Cancer Res 2005;11(11):3974–86.

[2] Miles DW, Chan A, Dirix LY, Cortes J, Pivot X, Tomczak P, Delozier T, Sohn JH, Provencher L, Puglisi F, Harbeck N, Steger GG, Schneeweiss A, Wardley AM, Chlistalla A, Romieu G. Phase III study of bevacizumab plus docetaxel compared with placebo plus docetaxel for the first-line treatment of human epidermal growth factor receptor 2-negative metastatic breast cancer. J Clin Oncol 2010;28(20):3239–47.

[3] Robert NJ, Dieras V, Glaspy J, Brufsky AM, Bondarenko I, Lipatov ON, Perez EA, Yardley DA, Chan SY, Zhou X, Phan SC, O'Shaughnessy J. RIBBON-1: randomized, double-blind, placebo-controlled, phase III trial of chemotherapy with or without bevacizumab for first-line treatment of human epidermal growth factor receptor 2-negative, locally recurrent or metastatic breast cancer. J Clin Oncol 2011;29(10):1252–60.

[4] Schwab LP, Peacock DL, Majumdar D, Ingels JF, Jensen LC, Smith KD, Cushing RC, Seagroves TN. Hypoxia inducible factor-1α promotes primary tumor growth and tumor-initiating cell activity in breast cancer. Breast Cancer Res 2012;14(1):R6.

[5] Mooring SR, Jin H, Devi NS, Jabbar AA, Kaluz S, Liu Y, Van Meir EG, Wang B. Design and synthesis of novel small-molecule inhibitors of the hypoxia inducible factor pathway. J Med Chem 2011;54(24):8471–89.

[6] Birner P, Schindl M, Obermair A, Plank C. Overexpression of hypoxia-inducible factor 1α is a marker for an unfavorable prognosis in early-stage invasive cervical cancer. Cancer Res 2000;60:4693–6.

[7] Trinh XB, Tjalma WA, Vermeulen PB, Van den Eynden G, Van der Auwera I, Van Laere SJ, Helleman J, Berns EM, Dirix LY, van Dam PA. The VEGF pathway and the AKT/mTOR/p70S6K1 signalling pathway in human epithelial ovarian cancer. Br J Cancer 2009;100(6):971–8.

[8] Karar J, Maity A. PI3K/AKT/mTOR pathway in angiogenesis. Front Mol Neurosci 2011;4:51.

[9] Rundhaug JE. Matrix metalloproteinases and angiogenesis. J Cell Mol Med 2005;9(2):267–85.

[10] Paduch R. The role of lymphangiogenesis and angiogenesis in tumor metastasis. Cell Oncol (Dordr) 2016;39(5):397–410.

[11] Miller K, Wang M, Gralow J, Dickler M, Cobleigh M, Perez EA, Shenkier T, Cella D, Davidson NE. Paclitaxel plus bevacizumab versus paclitaxel alone for metastatic breast cancer. N Engl J Med 2007;357(26):2666–76.

[12] FDA begins process to remove breast cancer indication from Avastin label 2010. Available from: http://www.fda.gov/NewsEvents/Newsroom/PressAnnouncements/2010/ucm237172.htm

[13] Hsu JY, Wakelee HA. Monoclonal antibodies targeting vascular endothelial growth factor: current status and future challenges in cancer therapy. Biodrugs 2009;23(5):289–304.

[14] Regeneron Pharmaceuticals Inc. Eylea Prescribing Information 2011. Available from: http://www.regeneron.com/eylea

[15] Sanofi-Aventis. A multinational, randomized, double-blind study, comparing the efficacy of aflibercept once every 2 weeks versus placebo in patients with metastatic colorectal cancer (MCRC) treated with irinotecan/5-FU combination (FOLFIRI) after failure of an oxaliplatin based regimen. Available from: http://clinicaltrials.gov/ct2/show/NCT00561470?term =velour&rank=1

[16] Herbst RS, Hong D, Chap L, Kurzrock R, Jackson E, Silverman JM, Rasmussen E, Sun YN, Zhong D, Hwang YC, Evelhoch JL, Oliner JD, Le N, Rosen LS. Safety, pharmacokinetics, and antitumor activity of AMG 386, a selective angiopoietin inhibitor, in adult patients with advanced solid tumors. J Clin Oncol 2009;27(21):3557–65.

[17] Amgen. A phase 3 randomized, double-blind, placebo-controlled, multicenter study of AMG 386 with paclitaxel and carboplatin as first-line treatment of subjects with FIGO stage III-IV epithelial ovarian, primary peritoneal or fallopian tube cancers. Available from: http://clinicaltrials. gov/ct2/show/NCT01493505?term=trinova-3&rank=1

[18] Spratlin JL, Cohen RB, Eadens M, Gore L, Camidge DR, Diab S, Leong S, O'Bryant C, Chow LQ, Serkova NJ, Meropol NJ, Lewis NL, Chiorean EG, Fox F, Youssoufian H, Rowinsky EK, Eckhardt SG. Phase I pharmacologic and biologic study of ramucirumab (IMC-1121B), a fully human immunoglobulin G1 monoclonal antibody targeting the vascular endothelial growth factor receptor-2. J Clin Oncol 2010;28(5):780–7.

[19] O'Sullivan Coyne G, Burotto M. Clinical experience with ramucirumab: outcomes in breast cancer. Expert Opin Biol Ther 2014;14(9):1351–60.

[20] Zhu AX, Park JO, Ryoo BY, Yen CJ, Poon R, Pastorelli D, Blanc JF, Chung HC, Baron AD, Pfiffer TE, Okusaka T, Kubackova K, Trojan J, Sastre J, Chau I, Chang SC, Abada PB, Yang L, Schwartz JD, Kudo M, and REACH Trial Investigators. Ramucirumab versus placebo as second-line treatment in patients with advanced hepatocellular carcinoma following first-line therapy with sorafenib (REACH): a randomised, double-blind, multicentre, phase 3 trial. Lancet Oncol 2015;16(7):859–70.

[21] Wagner S, Rothweiler F, Anhorn MG, Sauer D, Riemann I, Weiss EC, Katsen-Globa A, Michaelis M, Cinatl J Jr, Schwartz D, Kreuter J, von Briesen H, Langer K. Enhanced drug targeting by attachment of an anti αv integrin antibody to doxorubicin loaded human serum albumin nanoparticles. Biomaterials 2010;31(8):2388–98.

[22] Pfizer Labs Inc. Sutent Prescribing Information 2011. Available from: https://www.pfizerpro.com/product/sutent?source=google&HBX_ PK=s_sutent+prescribing+information&o=79635665|255968740|0&s kwid=43700000844048558

[23] Shirao K, Nishida T, Doi T, Komatsu Y, Muro K, Li Y, Ueda E, Ohtsu A. Phase I/II study of sunitinib malate in Japanese patients with gastrointestinal stromal tumor after failure of prior treatment with imatinib mesylate. Invest New Drugs 2010;28(6):866–75.

[24] Llovet JM, Ricci S, Mazzaferro V, Hilgard P, Gane E, Blanc JF, de Oliveira AC, Santoro A, Raoul JL, Forner A, Schwartz M, Porta C, Zeuzem S, Bolondi L, Greten TF, Galle PR, Seitz JF, Borbath I, Haussinger D, Giannaris T, Shan M, Moscovici M, Voliotis D, Bruix J, Sharp Investigators Study Group. Sorafenib in advanced hepatocellular carcinoma. N Engl J Med 2008;359(4):378–90.

[25] Bayer Healthcare Pharmaceuticals Inc. Nexavar (sorafenib) tablets. Available from: https://www.nexavar.com/home/

[26] Escudier B, Eisen T, Stadler WM, Szczylik C, Oudard S, Staehler M, Negrier S, Chevreau C, Desai AA, Rolland F, Demkow T, Hutson TE, Gore M, Anderson S, Hofilena G, Shan M, Pena C, Lathia C, Bukowski RM. Sorafenib for treatment of renal cell carcinoma: final efficacy and safety results of the phase III treatment approaches in renal cancer global evaluation trial. J Clin Oncol 2009;27(20):3312–8.

[27] Astra Zeneca Pharmaceuticals. Caprelsa prescriber information. Available from: http://www.accessdata.fda.gov/drugsatfda_docs/label/2014/ 022405s007lbl.pdf

[28] Wells SA Jr, Gosnell JE, Gagel RF, Moley J, Pfister D, Sosa JA, Skinner M, Krebs A, Vasselli J, Schlumberger M. Vandetanib for the treatment of patients with locally advanced or metastatic hereditary medullary thyroid cancer. J Clin Oncol 2010;28(5):767–72.

[29] Novartis. Votrient prescribing information. Available from: http://www. hcp.novartis.com/products/votrient/advanced-renal-cell-carcinoma/?sit e=PS0012854&source=01030&IRMASRC=None

[30] Sternberg CN, Davis ID, Mardiak J, Szczylik C, Lee E, Wagstaff J, Barrios CH, Salman P, Gladkov OA, Kavina A, Zarba JJ, Chen M, McCann L, Pandite L, Roychowdhury DF, Hawkins RE. Pazopanib in locally advanced or metastatic renal cell carcinoma: results of a randomized phase III trial. J Clin Oncol 2010;28(6):1061–8.

[31] Gril B, Palmieri D, Qian Y, Anwar T, Ileva L, Bernardo M, Choyke P, Liewehr DJ, Steinberg SM, Steeg PS. The B-Raf status of tumor cells may be a significant determinant of both antitumor and anti-angiogenic effects of pazopanib in xenograft tumor models. PLoS One 2011;6(10):e25625.

[32] Dvorak HF. Tumor stroma, tumor blood vessels, and antiangiogenesis therapy. Cancer J 2015;21(4):237–43.

[33] Maloney SL, Sullivan DC, Suchting S, Herbert JM, Rabai EM, Nagy Z, Barker J, Sundar S, Bicknell R. Induction of thrombospondin-1 partially mediates the anti-angiogenic activity of dexrazoxane. Br J Cancer 2009;101(6):957–66.

[34] Ruf W, Disse J, Carneiro-Lobo TC, Yokota N, Schaffner F. Tissue factor and cell signalling in cancer progression and thrombosis. J Thromb Haemost 2011;9(Suppl. 1):306–15.

[35] Collen A, Smorenburg SM, Peters E, Lupu F, Koolwijk P, Van Noorden C, van Hinsbergh VW. Unfractionated and low molecular weight heparin affect fibrin structure and angiogenesis in vitro. Cancer Res 2000;60(21): 6196–200.

[36] Elice F, Rodeghiero F, Falanga A, Rickles FR. Thrombosis associated with angiogenesis inhibitors. Best Pract Res Clin Haematol 2009;22(1):115–28.

[37] Davis PJ, Davis FB, Mousa SA. Thyroid hormone-induced angiogenesis. Curr Cardiol Rev 2009;5(1):12–6.

[38] Mousa SA, Yalcin M, Bharali DJ, Meng R, Tang HY, Lin HY, Davis FB, Davis PJ. Tetraiodothyroacetic acid and its nanoformulation inhibit thyroid hormone stimulation of non-small cell lung cancer cells in vitro and its growth in xenografts. Lung Cancer 2011;76(1):39–45.

[39] Srinivasan M, Rajabi M, Mousa SA. Nanobiomaterials in cancer therapy. In: Grumezescu A, editor. Nanobiomaterials in cancer therapy: applications of nanobiomaterials, vol. 7. Amsterdam: Elsevier; 2016. p. 57–89.

[40] Rajabi M, Srinivasan M, Mousa SA. Nanobiomaterials in drug delivery. In: Grumezescu A, editor. Nanobiomaterials in Drug Delivery: Applications of Nanobiomaterials, vol. 9. Amsterdam: Elsevier; 2016. p. 1–39.

[41] Celgene Corporation. Thalidomide package insert. Available from: http://www.thalomid.com/

[42] Lin AY, Brophy N, Fisher GA, So S, Biggs C, Yock TI, Levitt L. Phase II study of thalidomide in patients with unresectable hepatocellular carcinoma. Cancer 2005;103(1):119–25.

[43] McCollum AD, Wu B, Clark JW, Kulke MH, Enzinger PC, Ryan DP, Earle CC, Michelini A, Fuchs CS. The combination of capecitabine and thalidomide in previously treated, refractory metastatic colorectal cancer. Am J Clin Oncol 2006;29(1):40–4.

[44] Celgene Corporation. Revlimid prescribing information. Available from: http://www.revlimid.com/

[45] Weber DM, Chen C, Niesvizky R, Wang M, Belch A, Stadtmauer EA, Siegel D, Borrello I, Rajkumar SV, Chanan-Khan AA, Lonial S, Yu Z, Patin J, Olesnyckyj M, Zeldis JB, Knight RD. Multiple Myeloma Study I.

Lenalidomide plus dexamethasone for relapsed multiple myeloma in North America. N Engl J Med 2007;357(21):2133–42.

[46] Wicki A, Rochlitz C, Orleth A, Ritschard R, Albrecht I, Herrmann R, Christofori G, Mamot C. Targeting tumor-associated endothelial cells: Anti-VEGFR2 immunoliposomes mediate tumor vessel disruption and inhibit tumor growth. Clin Cancer Res 2012;18(2):454–64.

[47] Lim ZZ, Li JE, Ng CT, Yung LY, Bay BH. Gold nanoparticles in cancer therapy. Acta Pharmacol Sin 2011;32(8):983–90.

[48] Mukherjee S, Patra CR. Therapeutic application of anti-angiogenic nanomaterials in cancers. Nanoscale 2016;8(25):12444–70.

[49] Rajabi M, Mousa SA. Lipid nanoparticles and their application in nanomedicine. Curr Pharm Biotechnol 2016;17(8):662–72.

[50] Srinivasan M, Rajabi M, Mousa SA. Multifunctional nanomaterials and their applications in drug delivery and cancer therapy. Nanomaterials-Basel 2015;5(4):1690–703.

[51] Hui JZ, Al Zaki A, Tsourkas A. Improving nanoparticle delivery with anti-angiogenesis therapy. Nanomedicine 2012;7(7):949–50.

[52] Banerjee D, Harfouche R, Sengupta S. Nanotechnology-mediated targeting of tumor angiogenesis. Vasc Cell 2011;3(1):3.

[53] Yoncheva K, Momekov G. Antiangiogenic anticancer strategy based on nanoparticulate systems. Expert Opin Drug Deliv 2011;8(8):1041–56.

[54] Chen YJ, Wang XR, Liu T, Zhang DSZ, Wang YF, Gu HC, Di W. Highly effective antiangiogenesis via magnetic mesoporous silica-based siRNA vehicle targeting the VEGF gene for orthotopic ovarian cancer therapy. Int J Nanomed 2015;10:2579–94.

[55] Xu Y, Wen Z, Xu Z. Chitosan nanoparticles inhibit the growth of human hepatocellular carcinoma xenografts through an antiangiogenic mechanism. Anticancer Res 2009;29(12):5103–9.

[56] Bharali DJ, Yalcin M, Davis PJ, Mousa SA. Tetraiodothyroacetic acid-conjugated PLGA nanoparticles: a nanomedicine approach to treat drug-resistant breast cancer. Nanomedicine (Lond) 2013;8(12):1943–54.

[57] Yalcin M, Bharali DJ, Lansing L, Dyskin E, Mousa SS, Hercbergs A, Davis FB, Davis PJ, Mousa SA. Tetraidothyroacetic acid (tetrac) and tetrac nanoparticles inhibit growth of human renal cell carcinoma xenografts. Anticancer Res 2009;29(10):3825–31.

[58] Mousa SA, Bharali DJ. Nanotechnology-based detection and targeted therapy in cancer: nano-bio paradigms and applications. Cancers (Basel) 2011;3(3):2888–903.

[59] Bharali DJ, Mousa SA. Emerging nanomedicines for early cancer detection and improved treatment: Current perspective and future promise. Pharmacol Ther 2010;128(2):324–35.

CHAPTER 11

Application of Nanotechnology to Target Tumor Angiogenesis in Cancer Therapeutics

Dhruba J. Bharali, Mehdi Rajabi and Shaker A. Mousa

Contents

INTRODUCTION

Cancer continues to be a deadly disease in the United States and globally. According to the American Cancer Society, an estimated 1,685,210 new cancer cases are expected to be diagnosed and 595,690 people will die from cancer in the United States in 2016 [1]. Despite tremendous efforts by researchers, there have been only limited advances in cancer treatment over the past several decades. Most of the current diagnostic and therapeutic approaches to diagnose and treat cancer rely predominantly on invasive (i.e., biopsies, surgery) and nonspecific techniques, such as irradiation and chemotherapeutic agents. Therefore, it is imperative to look for alternative therapeutic modalities that can significantly improve the often dismal prognosis of this disease. Nanotechnology, or in this chapter "nanomedicine," is a potential replacement for conventional cancer therapy to address many of the challenges in current cancer

Anti-Angiogenesis Strategies in Cancer Therapies
http://dx.doi.org/10.1016/B978-0-12-802576-5.00011-5

treatment. Scientific and medical communities are making significant progress in cancer diagnosis and treatment, and there are many studies that use a nanomedicine approach to target tumor vasculature for inhibiting angiogenesis.

ANGIOGENESIS

Angiogenesis, the formation and propagation of new blood vessels, is the most important support mechanism for tumor growth and development. Eliminating the formation of blood vessels in the tumor vasculature means inhibiting tumor growth. It is well established that a tumor cannot grow beyond 1–2 mm in size without angiogenesis [2], and therefore if we can inhibit angiogenesis we can potentially inhibit growth of the tumor (Fig. 11.1). The major advantage of targeting angiogenesis to treat cancer lies in the better accessibility of a drug to the tumor vasculature rather than to the solid tumor mass. This important fact can potentially decrease the tumor drug resistance and at the same time increase efficacy of the drug. Most current therapeutic strategies intended to stop the progress of the tumor

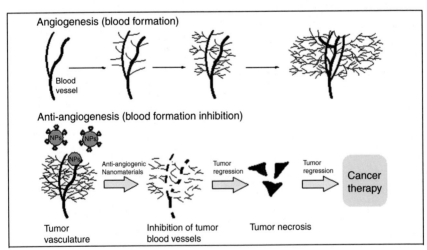

Figure 11.1 *Angiogenesis is the physiological process by which new blood vessels form from preexisting vessels. Nanomedicine using nanoparticles (NPs) is one approach to target anti-angiogenic factors and cause tumor regression.*

vascularization are at a preclinical stage, and only a handful of these strategies are emerging as clinical reality. A nanomedicine approach to target various anti-angiogenic factors is an alternative to conventional therapy to inhibit tumor angiogenesis [3–5] (Fig. 11.1).

INTEGRINS

Integrins play a vital role in tumor survival, migration and metastasis. Tumor cell expression of integrins is correlated with diseases in various tumor types (Fig. 11.2). Though αvβ3 and αvβ5 were the two integrins first targeted to inhibit tumor angiogenesis, now a wide array of integrins including α1β1, α2β1, α3β1, α4β1, α5β1, α6β1, αvβ3, αvβ5, and αvβ6 are targeted by researchers to suppress tumor angiogenesis.

Integrin αvβ3 Targeting with Nanoparticles

Accumulation of nanoparticles, in particular magnetic nanoparticles, on tumor vascularization has been shown in many studies. Magnetic resonance imaging (MRI) was used to determine the preferential accumulation of these αvβ3 targeting nanoparticles [6–9]. A 1998 study by Arap and coworkers [10] is one of the pioneering studies to demonstrate the feasibility of targeted chemotherapy tactics using an αv binding agent. They used an Arg-Gly-Asp (RGD) motif attached to doxorubicin to increase uptake of this chemotherapeutic drug. The efficacy of the doxorubicin

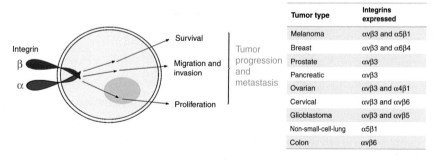

Tumor type	Integrins expressed
Melanoma	αvβ3 and α5β1
Breast	αvβ3 and α6β4
Prostate	αvβ3
Pancreatic	αvβ3
Ovarian	αvβ3 and α4β1
Cervical	αvβ3 and αvβ6
Glioblastoma	αvβ3 and αvβ5
Non-small-cell-lung	α5β1
Colon	αvβ6

Figure 11.2 *Tumor cell expression of the integrins is correlated with disease progression in various tumor types.*

was tested in breast cancer xenografts in nude mice. Since then numerous strategies including several nanoparticles-mediated $\alpha v \beta 3$ targeting agents containing different therapeutics have been tested [11–13]. Another notable study of doxorubicin delivery was performed by Murphy and coworkers [14]. They synthesized $\alpha v \beta 3$ targeting nanoparticles with the capacity to deliver doxorubicin to the tumor vasculature. These nanoparticles, made up of distearoylphosphatidylcholine (DSPC), cholesterol dioleoylphosphatidylethanolamine (DOPE), distearoylphosphatidylethanolamine (DSPE)-mPEG2000 along with RGD were able to incorporate doxorubicin successfully. The authors showed the capability of these nanoparticles to control metastasis of pancreatic cancer and renal cell carcinoma in orthotopic mouse models. The RGD-guided nanoparticles carrying doxorubicin to the tumor vascularization were able to increase the dose response of the drug up to 15-fold when compared to free doxorubicin. Thus, it can be anticipated that the targeted delivery of cytotoxic drugs like doxorubicin nanoparticles have the potential to decrease adverse side effects by limiting the drugs' distribution in the body and also have the capability to limit the tumor metastasis. Apart from these studies, there have been many studies performed in the last few years either to exploit the site-directed delivery of nanoparticles to the tumor neovascularization or to enhance the therapeutic benefit of the anti-cancer drugs. A list of these studies is in Table 11.1.

Integrin $\alpha v \beta 3$ Targeting with Tetrac Nanoformulation

For the last several years, our laboratory has been working on developing a nanoformulation conjugating tetraiodothyroacetic acid (tetrac) to the biodegradable polymer poly(lactide-co-glycolide) (PLGA). We have demonstrated that tetrac, a thyroid hormone analog, has anti-angiogenic properties that are relevant to the vascular supply of tumors [26,27]. Tetrac targets a plasma membrane receptor on integrin $\alpha v \beta 3$ [26–28]. However, in its free form tetrac can potentially enter the cell nucleus and thus has the potential to exert adverse genomic effects (when administered as an anti-cancer agent). Our nanomedicine approach of conjugating tetrac

Table 11.1 Examples of nanoparticles-mediated targeting of tumor angiogenesis therapeutics

Type of nanoparticles	Targeting moiety	Therapeutics	Imaging	Therapy	Animal model	References
Lipid based, containing gadolinium	$\alpha_v\beta_3$-integrin peptidomimetic antagonist	None	MRI	No	Rabbits implanted with Vx-2 tumors	[7]
Hollow gold nanospheres	Cyclic RGD peptide c(KRGDf)	Photothermal ablation (PTA)	PET	Yes	Both glioma and angiogenic blood vessels	[16]
Polyethylene glycol–polylactic acid (PEG–PLA)	None	TNP-470	None	Yes	Mice, corneal micropocket angiogenesis and intrasplenic model for induction of liver metastasis	[17]
Poly (lactide-co-glycolide) (PLGA)	None	Combretastatin-A4 and doxorubicin	None	Yes	Mice (B16/F10 melanomas or Lewis lung carcinoma)	[18]
Integrin-targeted nanoparticle	Integrin antagonist (Bis-T-PE-EDTA-IA)	None	Fluorescence microscopy	No	Mice, SCC 7 murine squamous cell carcinoma	[19]
Hexadentate-poly D,L-lactic acid-co-glycolic	None	PD98059, cisplatin	Fluorescence microscopy	Yes	Mice, melanoma-bearing	[20]

(Continued)

Table 11.1 Examples of nanoparticles-mediated targeting of tumor angiogenesis therapeutics (*cont.*)

Type of nanoparticles	Targeting moiety	Therapeutics	Imaging	Therapy	Animal model	References
Quantum dots	RGD peptides	None	PET/NIRF	No	Mice, U87MG tumor-bearing	[21]
Gold	Cyclic RGD peptides	None	Micro–SPECT/CT	No	Athymic mice with C6-induced tumors	[22]
PLGA	RGD peptides	Paclitaxel and combretastatin	None	Yes	Mice	[23]
Nano graphene oxide	TRC105, a monoclonal antibody	None	PET	No	Mice, 4T1 murine breast tumor-bearing	[24]
Iron oxide nano worms	Tumor-penetrating peptide iRGD	α–Helical amphipathic peptide $_D$[KLAKLAK]$_2$	MRI	Yes	Mice, orthotopic glioblastoma–bearing	[25]

Abbreviations: CT, Computed tomography; MRI, magnetic resonance imaging; NIRF, near-infrared fluorescence; PET, positron emission tomography; SPECT, single-photon emission computed tomography.

Source: Modified with permission of Springer: Bharali DJ, Mousa SA. Angiogenesis modulations in health and disease. Application of nanotechnology to prevent tumor angiogenesis for therapeutic benefit, 2013, p. 176–177, [Chapter 14] [15].

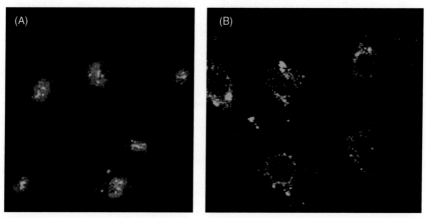

Figure 11.3 Confocal images showing the uptake of (A) Alexa Fluor labeled free thyroid hormone, (B) T-PLGA-NPs labeled with Alexa Fluor 488 dye; in human dermal microvascular endothelial cells (HDMEC) cells. *(Courtesy: Bharali et al. Nanomedicine, London) [29].*

to PLGA nanoparticles (T-PLGA-NPs) can overcome this problem by preventing the nanoparticles from entering the nucleus. This is primarily because the larger size of the nanoparticles prevents them from going into the nucleus (Fig. 11.3) [29]. At the same time, these nanoparticles achieve the targeting of tetrac to its receptor on plasma membrane integrin $\alpha v \beta 3$. This property of the nanoparticles enables us to use this nanofomulation as a therapeutic means to investigate the anti-angiogenic and anti-proliferative actions of tetrac via the extracellular domain of the integrin. These nanoformulations cause significant inhibition of angiogenesis in a chick chorioallantoic membrane (CAM) model of angiogenesis (Fig. 11.4) [29].

Recently we have done several studies in different tumor xenograft mouse models. In most of these studies, the nanoparticles showed anti-cancer efficacy either equivalent or superior to existing chemotherapeutic agents or to unmodified tetrac in different in vivo tumor models including renal cell carcinoma [30], medullary cell carcinoma [31], follicular cell carcinoma [32], and non-small lung cancer cells [33]. These T-PLGA-NPS have even been shown to be effective in inhibiting doxorubicin-resistant breast cancer tumors in a mouse model [29]. Based on our

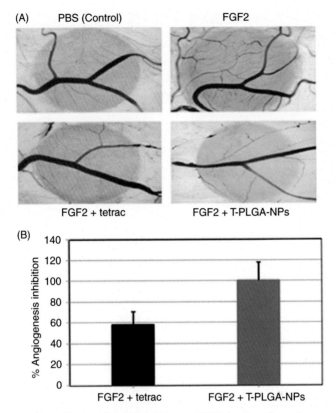

Figure 11.4 *The effects of T-PLGA-NPs on FGF2-induced angiogenesis measured by the CAM assay.* (A) Photomicrographs of representative CAMs treated with free tetrac or T-PLGA-NPs. CAMs were also treated with FGF2 or PBS as a positive and negative control, respectively. (B) Quantification of angiogenesis inhibition by tetrac versus T-PLGA-NPs. Data represents number of branch points and were normalized to the negative control, PBS. Data are expressed as percent inhibition of angiogenesis induced by FGF2 alone (means ± SEM), *$p \leq 0.01$. *(Courtesy: Bharali et al. Nanomedicine, London) [29]*.

preliminary studies, we propose that these nanoparticles can be used to treat a variety of chemo–resistant tumors in addition to resistant breast cancer. Another major advantage of this nano-formulation is its ability to incorporate various chemotherapeutic drugs in its polymeric network. Further, the $\alpha v \beta 3$ integrin targeting nanoformulations can transport and deliver additional anti-cancer agents in their nanoparticle component. We have encapsulated different chemotherapeutic drugs, such as cisplatin, paclitaxel, and doxorubicin for delivery at αvβ3 integrin-bearing cancers. The result is significantly improved tumor xenograft uptake of the chemotherapeutic agent and reduced systemic exposure to the drug. An example of the latter is that cisplatin neurotoxicity was eliminated in xenografted animals by encapsulation of cisplatin in T-PLGA-NPs [34].

GENE THERAPY DELIVERY WITH NANOPARTICLES

Delivering a therapeutic gene to inhibit angiogenesis via nanoparticles is another potential therapeutic approach for the inhibition of tumor growth. It is well established that nanoparticle-delivered genes are much easier to synthesize, are less toxic, and are safer than their "viral vector" counterparts [35,36]. A pioneering study by Hood and coworkers [37] incorporated an αvβ3 targeting moiety (the LM609 antibody) in lipid nanoparticles. These nanoparticles were capable of carrying a mutant Rag gene, ATP^{μ}-Raf-1. This gene was delivered via the nanoparticles to the tumor vasculature and interfered with the signaling cascades of two important angiogenic growth factors, basic fibroblast growth factor (bFGF) and vascular endothelial growth factor (VEGF). Pigment epithelium-derived factor (PEDF) gene therapy is another area of intense cancer research in inhibition of tumor angiogenesis. Yu and coworkers [38] developed COOH-PEG-PLGA-COOH (CPPC) nanoparticles loaded with the *PEDF* gene. These CPPC nanoparticles encapsulating the *PEDF* gene showed excellent cytotoxic effects on C26, A549, and HUVEC cell lines. Additionally, it was found that CPPC nanoparticles encapsulating *PEDF* gene can effectively suppress the growth of C26 tumor xenografts. Nanoparticles-mediated delivery of small interfering RNA (siRNA) can also be very useful to treat tumor angiogenesis by serving to knock down a gene responsible for tumor progression. In a study by Chen and coworkers [39], VEGF-siRNA was successfully encapsulated in mesoporous silica based nanoparticles (MSNs) with high loading efficiency. These VEGF-based silica nanoparticles carrying VEGF-siRNA showed remarkable tumor suppression in murine lung and ovarian cancer tumor models [39,40]. Apart from these examples, there are numerous reports showing the use of siRNA/short hairpin RNA (shRNA) targeting tumor vasculature [24,41–45] to inhibit angiogenesis. Results of many of these studies are promising.

CONCLUSIONS

Although some improvement has been made in clinical interruption of cancer angiogenesis, to date most studies are confined to preclinical settings. In our opinion, a systematic nanomedicine study in a preclinical model can be rapidly translated into a successful clinical outcome and holds the key to success of this approach of targeting/inhibiting tumor vasculature. Considering the huge potential of its therapeutic benefit, a nanomedicine approach to target tumor angiogenesis can be the next generation approach to cancer treatment. In summary, site-specific nanoparticles-mediated delivery of multiple anti-cancer drugs to the tumor vasculature is one of a number of unique properties that make the nanomedicine platform an attractive and current approach to inhibition of tumor angiogenesis.

REFERENCES

[1] American Cancer Society. Cancer Facts & Figures 2016 [cited 2016 July 8]. Available from: http://www.cancer.org/acs/groups/content/@ research/documents/document/acspc-047079.pdf

[2] Kohandel M, Kardar M, Milosevic M, Sivaloganathan S. Dynamics of tumor growth and combination of anti-angiogenic and cytotoxic therapies. Phys Med Biol 2007;52(13):3665–77.

[3] Rajabi M, Srinivasan M, Mousa SA. Nanobiomaterials in drug delivery. In: Grumezescu A, editor. Nanobiomaterials in drug delivery: applications of nanobiomaterials, vol. 9. Amsterdam: Elsevier; 2016. p. 1–39.

[4] Srinivasan M, Rajabi M, Mousa SA. Multifunctional nanomaterials and their applications in drug delivery and cancer therapy. Nanomaterials 2015;5(4):1690–703.

[5] Srinivasan M, Rajabi M, Mousa SA. Nanobiomaterials in cancer therapy. In: Grumezescu A, editor. Nanobiomaterials in cancer therapy: applications of nanobiomaterials, vol. 7. Amsterdam: Elsevier; 2016. p. 57–89.

[6] Sipkins DA, Cheresh DA, Kazemi MR, Nevin LM, Bednarski MD, Li KC. Detection of tumor angiogenesis in vivo by $\alpha v \beta 3$-targeted magnetic resonance imaging. Nat Med 1998;4(5):623–6.

[7] Winter PM, Caruthers SD, Kassner A, Harris TD, Chinen LK, Allen JS, Lacy EK, Zhang H, Robertson JD, Wickline SA, Lanza GM. Molecular imaging of angiogenesis in nascent Vx-2 rabbit tumors using a novel $\alpha v \beta 3$-targeted nanoparticle and 1.5 tesla magnetic resonance imaging. Cancer Res 2003;63(18):5838–43.

[8] Hu H, Arena F, Gianolio E, Boffa C, Di Gregorio E, Stefania R, Orio L, Baroni S, Aime S. Mesoporous silica nanoparticles functionalized with fluorescent and MRI reporters for the visualization of murine tumors overexpressing $\alpha v \beta 3$ receptors. Nanoscale 2016;8(13):7094–104.

[9] Hu Y, Li J, Yang J, Wei P, Luo Y, Ding L, Sun W, Zhang G, Shi X, Shen M. Facile synthesis of RGD peptide-modified iron oxide nanoparticles with ultrahigh relaxivity for targeted MR imaging of tumors. Biomater Sci 2015;3(5):721–32.

[10] Arap W, Pasqualini R, Ruoslahti E. Cancer treatment by targeted drug delivery to tumor vasculature in a mouse model. Science 1998;279(5349): 377–80.

[11] Yuan Y, Wang Z, Cai P, Liu J, Liao LD, Hong M, Chen X, Thakor N, Liu B. Conjugated polymer and drug co-encapsulated nanoparticles for chemo- and photo-thermal combination therapy with two-photon regulated fast drug release. Nanoscale 2015;7(7):3067–76.

[12] Tsiapa I, Efthimiadou EK, Fragogeorgi E, Loudos G, Varvarigou AD, Bouziotis P, Kordas GC, Mihailidis D, Nikiforidis GC, Xanthopoulos S, Psimadas D, Paravatou-Petsotas M, Palamaris L, Hazle JD, Kagadis GC. ^{99m}Tc-labeled aminosilane-coated iron oxide nanoparticles for molecular imaging of $\alpha v \beta 3$-mediated tumor expression and feasibility for hyperthermia treatment. J Colloid Interface Sci 2014;433:163–75.

[13] Xie H, Diagaradjane P, Deorukhkar AA, Goins B, Bao A, Phillips WT, Wang Z, Schwartz J, Krishnan S. Integrin $\alpha v \beta 3$-targeted gold nanoshells augment tumor vasculature-specific imaging and therapy. Int J Nanomed 2011;6:259–69.

[14] Murphy EA, Majeti BK, Barnes LA, Makale M, Weis SM, Lutu-Fuga K, Wrasidlo W, Cheresh DA. Nanoparticle-mediated drug delivery to tumor vasculature suppresses metastasis. Proc Natl Acad Sci USA 2008;105(27):9343–8.

[15] Bharali DJ, Mousa SA. Application of nanotechnology to prevent tumor angiogenesis for therapeutic benefit. In: Mousa SA, Davis PJ, editors. Angiogenesis modulations in health and disease. Netherlands: Springer; 2013. p. 173–80.

[16] Lu W, Melancon MP, Xiong C, Huang Q, Elliott A, Song S, Zhang R, Flores LG 2nd, Gelovani JG, Wang LV, Ku G, Stafford RJ, Li C. Effects of photoacoustic imaging and photothermal ablation therapy mediated by targeted hollow gold nanospheres in an orthotopic mouse xenograft model of glioma. Cancer Res 2011;71(19):6116–21.

[17] Benny O, Fainaru O, Adini A, Cassiola F, Bazinet L, Adini I, Pravda E, Nahmias Y, Koirala S, Corfas G, D'Amato RJ, Folkman J. An orally delivered small-molecule formulation with antiangiogenic and anticancer activity. Nat Biotechnol 2008;26(7):799–807.

[18] Sengupta S, Eavarone D, Capila I, Zhao G, Watson N, Kiziltepe T, Sasisekharan R. Temporal targeting of tumour cells and neovasculature with a nanoscale delivery system. Nature 2005;436(7050):568–72.

[19] Xie J, Shen Z, Li KC, Danthi N. Tumor angiogenic endothelial cell targeting by a novel integrin-targeted nanoparticle. Int J Nanomed 2007;2(3):479–85.

[20] Basu S, Harfouche R, Soni S, Chimote G, Mashelkar RA, Sengupta S. Nanoparticle-mediated targeting of MAPK signaling predisposes tumor to chemotherapy. Proc Natl Acad Sci USA 2009;106(19):7957–61.

[21] Cai W, Chen K, Li ZB, Gambhir SS, Chen X. Dual-function probe for PET and near-infrared fluorescence imaging of tumor vasculature. J Nucl Med 2007;48(11):1862–70.

[22] Morales-Avila E, Ferro-Flores G, Ocampo-Garcia BE, De Leon-Rodriguez LM, Santos-Cuevas CL, Garcia-Becerra R, Medina LA, Gomez-Olivan L. Multimeric system of ^{99m}Tc-labeled gold nanoparticles conjugated to c[RGDfK(C)] for molecular imaging of tumor $\alpha(v)\beta(3)$ expression. Bioconjug Chem 2011;22(5):913–22.

[23] Wang Z, Chui WK, Ho PC. Nanoparticulate delivery system targeted to tumor neovasculature for combined anticancer and antiangiogenesis therapy. Pharm Res 2011;28(3):585–96.

[24] Hong H, Yang K, Zhang Y, Engle JW, Feng L, Yang Y, Nayak TR, Goel S, Bean J, Theuer CP, Barnhart TE, Liu Z, Cai W. In vivo targeting and imaging of tumor vasculature with radiolabeled, antibody-conjugated nanographene. ACS Nano 2012;6(3):2361–70.

[25] Agemy L, Friedmann-Morvinski D, Kotamraju VR, Roth L, Sugahara KN, Girard OM, Mattrey RF, Verma IM, Ruoslahti E. Targeted nanoparticle enhanced proapoptotic peptide as potential therapy for glioblastoma. Proc Natl Acad Sci USA 2011;108(42):17450–5.

[26] Rebbaa A, Chu F, Davis FB, Davis PJ, Mousa SA. Novel function of the thyroid hormone analog tetraiodothyroacetic acid: a cancer chemosensitizing and anti-cancer agent. Angiogenesis 2008;11(3):269–76.

[27] Mousa SA, Bergh JJ, Dier E, Rebbaa A, O'Connor LJ, Yalcin M, Aljada A, Dyskin E, Davis FB, Lin HY, Davis PJ. Tetraiodothyroacetic acid, a small molecule integrin ligand, blocks angiogenesis induced by vascular endothelial growth factor and basic fibroblast growth factor. Angiogenesis 2008;11(2):183–90.

[28] Rajabi M, Sudha T, Darwish NH, Davis PJ, Mousa SA. Synthesis of MR-49, a deiodinated analog of tetraiodothyroacetic acid (tetrac), as a novel pro-angiogenesis modulator. Bioorg Med Chem Lett 2016;26(16):4112–6.

[29] Bharali DJ, Yalcin M, Davis PJ, Mousa SA. Tetraiodothyroacetic acid-conjugated PLGA nanoparticles: a nanomedicine approach to treat drug-resistant breast cancer. Nanomedicine 2013;8(12):1943–54.

[30] Yalcin M, Bharali DJ, Lansing L, Dyskin E, Mousa SS, Hercbergs A, Davis FB, Davis PJ, Mousa SA. Tetraidothyroacetic acid (tetrac) and tetrac nanoparticles inhibit growth of human renal cell carcinoma xenografts. Anticancer Res 2009;29(10):3825–31.

[31] Yalcin M, Dyskin E, Lansing L, Bharali DJ, Mousa SS, Bridoux A, Hercbergs AH, Lin HY, Davis FB, Glinsky GV, Glinskii A, Ma J, Davis PJ, Mousa SA. Tetraiodothyroacetic acid (tetrac) and nanoparticulate tetrac arrest growth of medullary carcinoma of the thyroid. J Clin Endocrinol Metab 2010;95(4):1972–80.

[32] Yalcin M, Bharali DJ, Dyskin E, Dier E, Lansing L, Mousa SS, Davis FB, Davis PJ, Mousa SA. Tetraiodothyroacetic acid and tetraiodothyroacetic acid nanoparticle effectively inhibit the growth of human follicular thyroid cell carcinoma. Thyroid 2010;20(3):281–6.

[33] Mousa SA, Yalcin M, Bharali DJ, Meng R, Tang HY, Lin HY, Davis FB, Davis PJ. Tetraiodothyroacetic acid and its nanoformulation inhibit thyroid hormone stimulation of non-small cell lung cancer cells in vitro and its growth in xenografts. Lung Cancer 2012;76(1):39–45.

[34] Sudha T, Bharali DJ, Yalcin M, Darwish NHE, Coskun MD, Keating KA, Lin HY, Davis PJ, Mousa SA. Targeted delivery of cisplatin to tumor xenografts via the nanoparticulate component of nano-diamino-tetrac. 2016, submitted.

[35] Bharali DJ, Klejbor I, Stachowiak EK, Dutta P, Roy I, Kaur N, Bergey EJ, Prasad PN, Stachowiak MK. Organically modified silica nanoparticles: a nonviral vector for in vivo gene delivery and expression in the brain. Proc Natl Acad Sci USA 2005;102(32):11539–44.

[36] Roy I, Ohulchanskyy TY, Bharali DJ, Pudavar HE, Mistretta RA, Kaur N, Prasad PN. Optical tracking of organically modified silica nanoparticles as DNA carriers: a nonviral, nanomedicine approach for gene delivery. Proc Natl Acad Sci USA 2005;102(2):279–84.

[37] Hood JD, Bednarski M, Frausto R, Guccione S, Reisfeld RA, Xiang R, Cheresh DA. Tumor regression by targeted gene delivery to the neovasculature. Science 2002;296(5577):2404–7.

[38] Yu T, Xu B, He L, Xia S, Chen Y, Zeng J, Liu Y, Li S, Tan X, Ren K, Yao S, Song X. Pigment epithelial-derived factor gene loaded novel COOH-PEG-PLGA-COOH nanoparticles promoted tumor suppression by systemic administration. Int J Nanomed 2016;11:743–59.

[39] Chen Y, Wang X, Liu T, Zhang DS, Wang Y, Gu H, Di W. Highly effective antiangiogenesis via magnetic mesoporous silica-based siRNA vehicle targeting the VEGF gene for orthotopic ovarian cancer therapy. Int J Nanomed 2015;10:2579–94.

[40] Chen Y, Gu H, Zhang DS, Li F, Liu T, Xia W. Highly effective inhibition of lung cancer growth and metastasis by systemic delivery of siRNA via multimodal mesoporous silica-based nanocarrier. Biomaterials 2014;35(38):10058–69.

[41] Lu ZX, Liu LT, Qi XR. Development of small interfering RNA delivery system using PEI-PEG-APRPG polymer for antiangiogenic vascular endothelial growth factor tumor-targeted therapy. Int J Nanomed 2011;6:1661–73.

[42] Hadj-Slimane R, Lepelletier Y, Lopez N, Garbay C, Raynaud F. Short interfering RNA (siRNA), a novel therapeutic tool acting on angiogenesis. Biochimie 2007;89(10):1234–44.

[43] Li YH, Shi QS, Du J, Jin LF, Du LF, Liu PF, Duan YR. Targeted delivery of biodegradable nanoparticles with ultrasound-targeted microbubble destruction-mediated hVEGF-siRNA transfection in human PC-3 cells in vitro. Int J Mol Med 2013;31(1):163–71.

[44] Schiffelers RM, Ansari A, Xu J, Zhou Q, Tang Q, Storm G, Molema G, Lu PY, Scaria PV, Woodle MC. Cancer siRNA therapy by tumor selective delivery with ligand-targeted sterically stabilized nanoparticle. Nucl Acids Res 2004;32(19):e149.

[45] Pille JY, Li H, Blot E, Bertrand JR, Pritchard LL, Opolon P, Maksimenko A, Lu H, Vannier JP, Soria J, Malvy C, Soria C. Intravenous delivery of anti-RhoA small interfering RNA loaded in nanoparticles of chitosan in mice: safety and efficacy in xenografted aggressive breast cancer. Hum Gene Ther 2006;17(10):1019–26.

CHAPTER 12

New Directions in Anti-Angiogenesis Research

Shaker A. Mousa and Paul J. Davis

Contents

INTRODUCTION

Extensive recent reviews have emphasized a spectrum of new directions in which anti-angiogenesis drug development may proceed [1,2]. Among the functional targets identified are hypoxia, tumor-promoting inflammation, tumor cell metabolism and acidosis, and endothelial cell migration. Certain intracellular signaling pathways critical to angiogenesis have repeatedly been stressed recently as targets, and these include Notch receptors/ligands and Eph receptors [1]. Anti-angiogenesis is also achieved with antagonism of endogenous vascular growth factors and disordering of the function of cell surface receptors for these factors, for example, interrupting modulatory crosstalk of such receptors and other plasma membrane proteins, such as the extracellular domain of integrin αvβ3. These factors and processes have been examined in a number of the chapters of this book. We review here in brief

Anti-Angiogenesis Strategies in Cancer Therapies
http://dx.doi.org/10.1016/B978-0-12-802576-5.00012-7

our speculations about new directions in which anti-angiogenesis research will proceed in the foreseeable future.

PROJECTIONS

Vascular Growth Factors

We project that previously unrecognized protein growth factors or isoforms of growth factors that are angiogenesis-relevant will be identified. An example of this direction in research is the vascular endothelial growth factor (VEGF) family that we now know contains isoforms VEGF-A through VEGF-E and placental growth factor (PlGF) [3]. Newly identified proangiogenic factors become biopharmaceutical targets of new antibodies or their signaling pathways are analyzed for specific inhibition by pharmacologic approaches. Models or clinical settings in which such new factors may be identified include spontaneous vascular malformations and in organ remodeling, such as that which occurs in the wake of ischemic damage. Existing biological products not previously appreciated to have angiogenic properties may be shown to promote angiogenesis and thus become targets of anti-angiogenic pharmacology. Examples of such biological products are melatonin [4] and lipocalin 2 (Lcn2; NGAL) [5]—now recognized to influence VEGF production—and the contribution of testosterone to revascularization of the postinfarcted heart [6]. The proangiogenic qualities of erythropoietin are now appreciated [7]. Targeting these products may be immunologic or may be directed at known receptor sites for these factors. With regard to melatonin, are the G protein-coupled receptors (MT1, MT2) linked to classical melatonin activities also involved in angiogenesis? Or are they previously unrecognized sites, such as we have found on a plasma membrane integrin for thyroid hormone, sex steroids or the stilbene, resveratrol (see next section on Integrin $\alpha v\beta 3$ and Growth Factors)? Antibodies to the integrin or Arg-Gly-Asp (RGD) peptides recognized by certain integrins may be prototypes of anti-angiogenic agents for such sites.

Integrin αvβ3 and Growth Factors

That crosstalk exists between integrin αvβ3 and nearby VEGF and basic fibroblast growth factor (bFGF) receptors on the cell surface is widely known. Such crosstalk at the cell surface or in or immediately beneath the plasma membrane may be a function of the binding of extracellular matrix (ECM) proteins by the integrin or messaging from within the cell (inside-out signaling). We have described on αvβ3 the existence of specific, high-affinity receptors for small endogenous ligands. These molecules include thyroid hormone [8], and the receptor for thyroid hormone on αvβ3 modifies interactions of VEGF and bFGF with their growth factor-specific cell surface receptors. Depending on the nature of the thyroid hormone analog bound to the integrin, the latter may generate pro- or anti-angiogenic signals. Testosterone and a steroid-like polyphenol, resveratrol, also have specific receptors on αvβ3. Is the testosterone receptor here where androgen stimulates the revascularization in the heart as described earlier? If so, the receptor becomes an anti-angiogenesis target. Resveratrol is an anti-angiogenic stilbene that acts to reduce VEGF production in human peritoneal mesothelial cell-dependent angiogenesis [9]. Interestingly, other stilbenes may be proangiogenic. Is this site where resveratrol initiates its anti-angiogenic activity, and can the resveratrol be pharmacologically packaged as an anti-angiogenic agent to target its receptor site on αvβ3? Estrogen has nongenomic actions that by definition do not primarily involve nuclear estrogen receptors, such as ERα. Such nongenomic actions may begin at the plasma membrane and, via these nonnuclear receptors, estrogen is known to modulate angiogenesis [10]. X-ray crystallographic modeling of the extracellular domain of integrin αvβ3 has revealed the presence of an estrogen-binding site [11] that is a candidate site for initiation of the proangiogenic action of estrogen. This site may be subject to pharmacologic blockade to eliminate the estrogen effect on blood vessel formation.

Transduction of Growth Factor Signals

Transduction of signals from pro- and anti-angiogenic factors expressed at their plasma membrane receptors has been well-characterized. The signal transduction process related to angiogenesis that is initiated by certain small molecules at $\alpha v\beta 3$ has also been defined and has revealed some novel features. The thyroid hormone receptor on $\alpha v\beta 3$ has two binding domains and one of these activates mitogen–activated protein kinase (MAPK; extracellular–regulated kinase 1/2, ERK 1/2) and the other stimulates phosphatidylinositol 3-kinase (PI3-K) activity (see Chapter 7). The domains recognize specific thyroid hormone analogs and can induce either pro- or anti-angiogenesis, depending on the ligand. Downstream of the integrin, these signal transducing pathways have discrete effects on transcription of specific genes. For example, usually suppressed expression of the tumor anti-angiogenic thrombospondin 1 (*TSP1*) gene [12] can be stimulated by a tetraiodothyroacetic acid (tetrac) formulation that acts at $\alpha v\beta 3$. Tetrac is a thyroid hormone analog that blocks actions of proangiogenic L-thyroxine (T_4), and this is a novel mechanism by which a thyroid hormone derivative can promote anti-angiogenesis. The activation by thyroid hormone—3, 5, 3'-triiodo-L-thyronine (T_3), but not T_4—of PI3-K at its $\alpha v\beta 3$ receptor leads downstream to expression of the hypoxia-inducible factor-1α (*HIF-1α*) gene [13] that is relevant to angiogenesis (see next section on Hypoxia). Tetrac formulations block this proangiogenic action of T_3 and are, again, anti-angiogneic. Such a signal transduction model may be relevant to the actions of other small molecules at angiogenesis–related receptors on the integrin. An $\alpha v\beta 3$-MAPK signaling pathway is also exploited by nonneuronal nicotinic acetylcholine receptors (AChRs), specifically $\alpha 7$ AChRs, that induce angiogenesis. Whether there are interactions of thyroid hormone and AChR–mediated actions is not yet known. However, nicotine, acting via an AChR, causes T_3 generation in brain via deiodination of T_4 (deiodinase 2, D2) [14]. This suggests that the proangiogenic activity of nicotine may relate to thyroid hormone.

Hypoxia

Hypoxia is an extraordinarily well-documented proangiogenic stimulus. The process is HIF-1α-dependent. Thus, agents demonstrated in the future to promote expression of the *HIF-1α* gene will be proangiogenic. Melatonin, lipocalin 2, and testosterone are, as discussed earlier, known to stimulate neovascularization. These factors also cause tissue accumulation of HIF-1α in cancers and may also do so in the process of remodeling of nonmalignant tissues. Estrogen is coupled to induction of *HIF-1α* gene expression by a complex nongenomic signal transduction pathway in breast cancer cells and this is presumptively linked to angiogenesis [15].

Inflammation-Related Signaling

New blood vessel formation accompanies the inflammatory process and the latter may also be a source of newly identified proangiogenic factors in the future. Examples of proinflammatory cytokines that are known to be proangiogenic are interleukin-8 (IL-8) in the context of cancer [16] and IL-18 in rheumatoid arthritis [17]. Among the chemokines that induce intratumoral angiogenesis are CCL3 and its specific receptor, CCR5 [18]. Thus, anti-angiogenic pharmaceutical design in oncology should consider contributions of cytokines and chemokines. Acting via integrin $\alpha v \beta 3$, tetrac formulations mentioned earlier may suppress transcription of certain chemokines and cytokines [19,20], but CCL3 and IL-8 have not been shown as yet to be subject to this regulation.

CONCLUSIONS

The earlier discussion has identified a number of areas of blood vessel biology in which new anti-angiogenic factors may be sought or to which novel anti-angiogenic drugs may be directed. As was noted at the outset of this discussion, there are a substantial number of targets and some of these have multiple downstream effects. Single target–single action therapeutic strategies in angiogenesis have been shown to be of limited utility. Net angiogenesis in a given tissue or model setting is the algebraic sum of pro- and anti-angiogenic factors present, and attacking a single factor when there is redundancy of factors and control mechanisms is unlikely to be clinically successful.

We have reviewed here the prospects of developing drugs that are anti-angiogenic by multiple mechanisms. Certain tyrosine kinase inhibitors are examples of currently available anti-cancer agents that may desirably disorder functioning of more than one vascular growth factor receptor (see Chapter 8). But the redundancy in tumor cells of control mechanisms for angiogenesis remains clinically defeating. Regulation of angiogenesis from integrin $\alpha v\beta 3$ includes multiple vascular growth factor genes and vascular growth factor receptor genes, and this has promise in preclinical studies. Are there other integrins or other plasma membrane proteins with similar arrays of growth factor functions relevant to angiogenesis? No matter the molecular strategy of anti-angiogenesis in the setting of cancer, clinical desirability remains paramount of targeted delivery of anti-angiogenic agents to cancer cells and to sites of tumor-related angiogenesis.

ACKNOWLEDGMENT

The authors appreciate the generous investment of Richard C. Liebich in much of the work reported in references 8, 11, 12 and 13 included in this review.

REFERENCES

[1] Khan KA, Bicknell R. Anti-angiogenic alternatives to VEGF blockade. Clin Exp Metastasis 2016;33(2):197–210.
[2] Wang Z, Dabrosin C, Yin X, Fuster MM, Arreola A, Rathmell WK, Generali D, Nagaraju GP, El-Rayes B, Ribatti D, Chen YC, Honoki K, Fujii H, Georgakilas AG, Nowsheen S, Amedei A, Niccolai E, Amin A, Ashraf SS, Helferich B, Yang X, Guha G, Bhakta D, Ciriolo MR, Aquilano K, Chen S, Halicka D, Mohammed SI, Azmi AS, Bilsland A, Keith WN, Jensen LD. Broad targeting of angiogenesis for cancer prevention and therapy. Semin Cancer Biol 2015;35:S224–43.
[3] Clauss M. Molecular biology of the VEGF and the VEGF receptor family. Semin Thromb Hemost 2000;26(5):561–9.

[4] Alvarez-Garcia V, Gonzalez A, Alonso-Gonzalez C, Martinez-Campa C, Cos S. Regulation of vascular endothelial growth factor by melatonin in human breast cancer cells. J Pineal Res 2013;54(4):373–80.

[5] Yang J, McNeish B, Butterfield C, Moses MA. Lipocalin 2 is a novel regulator of angiogenesis in human breast cancer. FASEB J 2013;27(1):45–50.

[6] Chen YP, Fu L, Han Y, Teng YQ, Sun JF, Xie RS, Cao JX. Testosterone replacement therapy promotes angiogenesis after acute myocardial infarction by enhancing expression of cytokines HIF-1a, SDF-1a and VEGF. Eur J Pharmacol 2012;684(1–3):116–24.

[7] Ribatti D. Erythropoietin and tumor angiogenesis. Stem Cells Dev 2010;19(1):1–4.

[8] Davis PJ, Davis FB, Mousa SA, Luidens MK, Lin HY. Membrane receptor for thyroid hormone: physiologic and pharmacologic implications. Annu Rev Pharmacol Toxicol 2011;51:99–115.

[9] Mikula-Pietrasik J, Kuczmarska A, Kucinska M, Murias M, Wierzchowski M, Winckiewicz M, Staniszewski R, Breborowicz A, Ksiazek K. Resveratrol and its synthetic derivatives exert opposite effects on mesothelial cell-dependent angiogenesis via modulating secretion of VEGF and IL-8/CXCL8. Angiogenesis 2012;15(3):361–76.

[10] Kim KH, Bender JR. Membrane-initiated actions of estrogen on the endothelium. Mol Cell Endocrinol 2009;308(1–2):3–8.

[11] Lin HY, Cody V, Davis FB, Hercbergs AA, Luidens MK, Mousa SA, Davis PJ. Identification and functions of the plasma membrane receptor for thyroid hormone analogues. Discov Med 2011;11(59):337–47.

[12] Glinskii AB, Glinsky GV, Lin HY, Tang HY, Sun M, Davis FB, Luidens MK, Mousa SA, Hercbergs AH, Davis PJ. Modification of survival pathway gene expression in human breast cancer cells by tetraiodothyroacetic acid (tetrac). Cell Cycle 2009;8(21):3562–70.

[13] Lin HY, Sun M, Tang HY, Lin C, Luidens MK, Mousa SA, Incerpi S, Drusano GL, Davis FB, Davis PJ. L-Thyroxine vs. 3,5,3'-triiodo-L-thyronine and cell proliferation: activation of mitogen-activated protein kinase and phosphatidylinositol 3-kinase. Am J Physiol Cell Physiol 2009;296(5):C980–91.

[14] Gondou A, Toyoda N, Nishikawa M, Yonemoto T, Sakaguchi N, Tokoro T, Inada M. Effect of nicotine on type 2 deiodinase activity in cultured rat glial cells. Endocr J 1999;46(1):107–12.

[15] Sudhagar S, Sathya S, Lakshmi BS. Rapid non-genomic signalling by 17β-oestradiol through c-Src involves mTOR-dependent expression of HIF-1α in breast cancer cells. Br J Cancer 2011;105(7):953–60.

[16] Waugh DJ, Wilson C. The interleukin-8 pathway in cancer. Clin Cancer Res 2008;14(21):6735–41.

[17] Volin MV, Koch AE. Interleukin-18: a mediator of inflammation and angiogenesis in rheumatoid arthritis. J Interferon Cytokine Res 2011;31(10):745–51.

[18] Wu Y, Li YY, Matsushima K, Baba T, Mukaida N. CCL3-CCR5 axis regulates intratumoral accumulation of leukocytes and fibroblasts and promotes angiogenesis in murine lung metastasis process. J Immunol 2008;181(9):6384–93.

[19] Davis PJ, Glinsky GV, Lin HY, Incerpi S, Davis FB, Mousa SA, Tang HY, Hercbergs A, Luidens MK. Molecular mechanisms of actions of formulations of the thyroid hormone analogue, tetrac, on the inflammatory response. Endocr Res 2013;38(2):112–8.

[20] Davis P, Glinsky G, Lin H, Mousa S. Actions of thyroid hormone analogues on chemokines. J Immunol Res 2016;2:1–7.

INDEX